The Psychology of Cancer

The Psychology of Cancer

Briefings for prevention and survival

Peter Lambley, PhD

Macdonald

A Macdonald Book

Copyright © Peter Lambley 1986

First published in Great Britain in 1987
by Macdonald & Co (Publishers) Ltd

Lambley, Peter
    The psychology of cancer.
    1. Cancer — Psychological aspects   2. Cancer
    — Social aspects
    I. Title
    616.99'4'0019   RC262

ISBN 0-356-10513-X

Typeset by Leaper & Gard Ltd, Bristol
Printed in Great Britain by
Redwood Burn Limited,
Bound at the Dorstel Press

Macdonald & Co (Publishers) Ltd
Greater London House
Hampstead Road
London NW1 7QX
A BPCC plc Company

In loving memory of my father,
Jack Lambley

Contents

Introduction   9

Chapter 1 Understanding Cancer   13

Chapter 2 Cancer and Personality   30

Chapter 3 A New Psychology of Cancer   45

Chapter 4 The Psychology of the Common Cancers   79

Chapter 5 Preventing Cancer   126

Chapter 6 Surviving Cancer   158

Final Word   194

Bibliography and Reading Notes   196

References   205

Index   231

ACKNOWLEDGEMENTS

A number of doctors, nurses, patients, researchers, hospitals and universities have provided help and advice over the past five years and I thank them all. In particular I thank the following for arranging visits and interviews, sending notes and research papers or otherwise communicating their thoughts to me:

Dr Godfrey Mdingi, Mr H. Hague, Dr C. Thomas, Dr Barbara Felton, Prof. A. Kazdin, Prof. David Reiss, Cancer Counselling & Research Centre, Prof. David Spiegel, Dr J. Marmor, Dr J. Holland, Dr Donna Funch, Dr R. Post, Dr Steven Locke, Prof. R. Ader, Dr J. Stephen Heisel, Dr R.S. Paffenberger, Dr Richard Berg, Dr W. Redd, Dr A. Forbes, Mrs L. Howe, Mr D. Fare, Mrs B. Hickman, Dr G. Maguire, Dr S. Greer, Prof. M. Wirsching, Dr A. Sellschop, Dr K. Jonasch, Dr H. Becker, Dr K. Foerster, Prof. F. Meerwein, Dr A. Zeigler, The Dutch Cancer Institute, Dr Luigi Valera, Prof. L. Keltingas-Jarvinen, Prof. K. Achte, The Psychiatric Clinic, University of Helsinki, Oncology Department, University of Odense, Kay Baltrop, Dr H. Steckelweh, Kester Berwick, D.L. Baider, Dr C. Margarey, Psychosomatic Clinic, Ruprecht-Karls University.

The ideas and opinions expressed in this book however except where clearly stated are solely my own responsibility and do not necessarily reflect the opinions of any of the above.

A special thanks to my old friend and colleague, Dr John King of Grooteschur Hospital. His ability to think creatively about cancer inspired many of my ideas at a time when few specialists recognised the importance of behaviour in the development of cancer. I am also deeply indebted to my wife Dorrian for the care and attention with which she has undertaken research and provided ideas for this book. We are both indebted to our secretary Jill Case without whose efforts the vast correspondence and typing tasks involved would never have been completed. Lastly, many thanks to Lana Odell my editor for much valuable and constructive advice.

INTRODUCTION

There is a rich psychological tradition running through the history of medicine. Over the centuries many conditions were thought to have strong psychological components and from very early on people who were predisposed to certain moods, who got easily depressed for instance, were ear-marked as candidates for a wide range of diseases. Cancer was one of these — so much so that by the nineteenth century, few textbooks appeared on the subject without copious reference being made to the psychological and emotional factors then thought to be involved in cancer. Unfortunately, no matter how much doctors believed the origins of cancer lay in the personality of the victim, they and families of cancer victims were seldom able to offer more than sympathy and kind words. It was surgery that offered the more immediate and practical help for cancer sufferers, and as surgical procedures improved — which they did in the nineteenth century — the rich psychological tradition in cancer quickly evaporated. Surgeons rather than physicians, psychologists, psychiatrists, or even general practitioners, became the key figures involved in cancer diagnosis and treatment. Cancer was seen as unquestionably a medical or organic problem with little or no room for psychology or the mind in its causation. Surgery has been the treatment of choice ever since and, indeed, remains the only means of preventing imminent death in many advanced cancers.

With all this emphasis on organic causes and the obvious power of surgical procedures, the role of the mind and emotions in cancer could easily have dwindled to a mere footnote in medical history. However, the psychological tradition in cancer did not disappear. For a time it remained dormant, kept up mainly by those on the fringes of medical practice. Faith healers, herbalists and the like, along with a number of unorthodox doctors, held firm to a belief in the power of mind over matter. They cared largely for those who were given up as hopeless cases by their surgeons — or who had not been helped by more orthodox treatments.

Periodically, too, as the new disciplines of psychology and psychiatry developed, a prominent psychologist or psychiatrist would offer interesting theories about the links between mind and cancer. Freud was one such, Wilhelm Reich another. Neither inspired much interest outside the ranks of their own followers and schools of thought; Freud himself died of cancer and Reich ended his days in an asylum, many of his ideas discredited.

Gradually, though, the value of scientific psychiatry and psychology began to gain popularity. After the Second World War researchers started to dig deeper into the causes of cancer with studies — some of them long-term, spanning thirty years — designed to identify the psychological and behavioural characteristics of people likely to develop cancer. Over time other researchers provided the first hard evidence that stress, lifestyle and personality played important roles in the development of cancer. Other studies indicated that psychological factors also play a role in cancer treatments; cancer victims can be encouraged to take better care of themselves and improve their chances of survival by adjusting their emotional attitudes. People who survive cancer are now known to have different psychological profiles from those who do not.

Also in the post-war years researchers in new medical disciplines like psychoneurology (the study of how the mind is linked to the nervous system) and immunology (how the body protects itself from disease) were unearthing just how closely the mind and the body interrelate. In the process these disciplines have created a new awareness that how a person thinks and feels and how he or she behaves are intricately related to body states and to whether or not they contract diseases like cancer.

Now, in the late 1980s, the sciences of psychology and human behaviour are well on the way to making a comeback in cancer research. Roughly a hundred years from when the mind and personality all but disappeared from cancer textbooks, we are seeing a renewed interest in mental phenomena by the medical profession. It comes at an opportune time. Despite the enormous amounts of money and energy spent on research and despite the obvious achievements made in treatment, cancer remains an enigma. Surgery, radiation and drug treatments have progressed remarkably, greatly improving chances of survival, especially if cancer is diagnosed early. But complete cure still cannot be guaranteed; prolonging life is the best that can be hoped for. Screening techniques, like routine breast and cervical examinations, have helped in early diagnosis and cut down on the number of fatalities from these cancers. But they have made little contribution to lowering the actual incidence of cancer; cervical cancer rates are as high as ever and other forms of cancer are on the increase — lung cancer, for example, is now as prevalent in women as it used to be in men. Medicine is still some way from fully understanding cancer and, on the face of it, seems no nearer to preventing it. Perhaps it is not surprising that many patients are turning to alternative therapies to try to fill the gaps left by standard medical treatment.

Could it be that the psychology of cancer would help to broaden the base of purely medical approaches to cancer treatment? Could a well-founded psychology of cancer help us to go on the offensive and develop effective cancer-prevention strategies? I believe that the answer to both these questions is 'yes' and that we are on the brink of a revolution in our thinking about the role of human behaviour in cancer.

The Psychology of Cancer is designed to present the reader with an up-to-date look at the fascinating new ideas about cancer that are gradually emerging in medical psychology and related fields. This is not a technical book. It is written to make the ordinary person aware of what cancer is, how it is treated and, above all, how the new psychology of cancer can help sufferers improve their chances of survival. Additionally it takes a long, hard look at how we as individuals can prevent cancer long before pre-cancerous changes occur in the body — not simply by advocating such things as giving up smoking, but in specifying the states of mind and habits of behaviour that lead to increased cancer risk in the first place, and outlining what immediate preventive steps can be taken.

Above all, this is a book about how people have survived cancer; case histories help illuminate research findings in a way relevant to day-to-day living. The book also tries to put the often confusing mass of evidence about cancer into a commonsense, easily understood framework that readers can use to their own advantage. It is aimed primarily at cancer victims, but if you are worried about cancer and your own future, there is much that will interest you. If you know someone with cancer and would like to help, this book contains useful insights to guide you in your approach.

Cancer is a very serious disease, but we are now beginning to realize that we can do far more to help ourselves than was previously thought. In fact, effective cancer prevention is now a very real possibility. This book tries to explain why.

CHAPTER 1
Understanding Cancer

When we think about cancer, unlike most illnesses, a bewildering range of emotions is invoked. We may not feel cheerful about strokes or heart attacks, but we know they are not necessarily fatal and often, if the right steps are taken, a person can survive and go on to resume a full life. The threat of cancer is different; for many people, it holds terror and little hope of survival. These attitudes affect doctors and nurses as well, especially if they have little to do with cancer patients. In fact, until the 1960s it was generally accepted in medical circles that it was best *not* to tell patients when they had cancer. Though attitudes have changed, recent evidence still suggests that doctors' *emotional* attitude to cancer dictates their approach to this question rather than a full understanding of research evidence.

When something is as distressing as this, we tend to turn away from it and cut off. We hope it will go away, that it will never happen to us or that one day, we will open the newspaper and read that a cure has been discovered. In any event, we avoid having a proper look at cancer. Left thus to the more primitive recesses of our minds, the idea of cancer becomes a dark, devouring monster and every snippet of fearful news is auto-

13

matically filed away, adding to its mystery. Most people hold
intense and highly emotional beliefs about cancer while, in fact,
seldom knowing the first thing about the disease. What does it
look like? Does it smell? Does it hurt? We'd rather not know.

Let's start this chapter by reviewing the basic facts about
cancer. Knowing one's enemy is half the battle won; looking at
cancer fairly and squarely means beginning to appreciate that
growths, benign and cancerous, are part and parcel of everyday
life. Cancer can take twenty years to develop to the size of a
small pea. The advantage of arming yourself with information
about cancer now gives you the opportunity to do something
about it before it's too late.

GROWTHS

The word *cancer* is of Latin origin and means a crab. The Greek
for the astrological sign of the crab is *karkino** (or carcinoma)
and both have been in use for many centuries to describe the
visible form of cancer on the skin, that of an unhealing ulcer. Its
slow and tenacious motion is reminiscent of those of a crab.
Cancer has been with us for a long time; tumours have been
found in the remains of neolithic man and in Egyptian
mummies. Most of the ancient civilizations of the world knew it
as a serious medical problem.

The basic component of cancer is a *tumour* or a *growth*.
What exactly are these? The body is made up of millions of *cells*
of different kinds, but all have in common the fact that they
grow to a certain size and level of activity, determined by the
kind of cell they are. These cells also have a set life; when they
age or are damaged, they die and are replaced by exact copies
(clones) which carry on their work. Sometimes the process of
creating new cells goes awry and too many are made. At the
same time these new cells are inferior, immature versions of the
original cells. In any given area this new mass (neoplasm) of
immature or abnormal cells constitutes a growth or tumour;

*The word crab in current Greek use is *kavouras*, but the astrological crab has
always been *karkinos*.

they may crowd out the healthier cells and form their own mass, or may coexist with healthy cells.

This growth is not yet a cancer. It's purely a growth, and the body can cope with quite a variety of small growths so long as they stay localized and *benign*. Warts and moles are benign growths, as are cysts; they can be classified as benign because they are very similar to healthy cells (i.e. not so badly matched) and do not invade the tissue around them. They may, of course be harmful if they get in the way of important body functions — a cyst in the eye, for example, can impede vision, or a benign tumour may push or squeeze vital organs or blood vessels — but by and large these are rare occurrences, and they do not do their damage by eating their way into other organs or tissue. Cancerous or *malignant* growths, however, are characterized by precisely the opposite activities; not satisfied with growing in their own space, they invade and destroy other tissue and cells around them. It is by *spreading* that cancer does its damage, first in the local area around the primary site and then through the infiltration of cancer cells into the blood, lymph glands and other parts of the body.

In all, then, there are three basic kinds of growths: benign, malignant (cancerous) and those that cannot easily be classed as either — intermediate growths. The last can best be defined as growths which appear cancerous and do invade local tissue, but do not metastasize, i.e. spread through the body. We can include in this category cancerous growths that may lie dormant for years before doing any harm, and growths that suddenly stop spreading. Classifying growths is not a simple cut and dried matter; it is quite complicated because cell behaviour is governed by a number of interlinked body processes.

The millions of cells in the body each have a specific job to do depending where they are. The skin is composed of cells, so too is the liver, bone marrow and, of course, the blood. We can divide the body into roughly three kinds of cell tissue: *epithelium*, *connective* and *lymph*. *Epithelium* tissue is the substance of your skin, the internal linings of your body, the membranes, glands and so, on. *Connective* tissue is found in the body support structure — the bones, fibres and so on. *Lymph* cells make up the substances of the blood, bone marrow etc.

Each of these different types of cell have a different function and relationship to the body's internal support systems; cells in the liver, for example, are fed, controlled and act in different ways from the cells on the skin of, say, your arms. Even cells of the same type can have different functions depending where they are; the epithelial cells on your arms do not allow substances to pass through them easily (skin really *is* waterproof), but the same kind of cells also line the air sacs inside your lungs and their main task is to allow substances (like oxygen) to pass through quickly.

So you can see that how a cell behaves depends on where it is, on the systems that service and support it, and its relationship to external, environmental events. Much the same is true of growths. How fast a tumour grows, whether or not it remains in the intermediate stage, whether or not it spreads (and how much) will clearly depend in large part on a mixture of all these factors. When cancers form in epithelium tissue we call them *carcinomas*; when they form in connective tissue they are called *sarcomas* and when they form in lymph cells we call them *lymphomas* or *leukaemias*. All are cancers and all act in similar ways at the *cellular* level, but how they appear and the effects they have differ according to the factors I have outlined above.

You are now in a position to recognize something very significant: cancer is not just one disease except in the simple sense that cancer cells all behave in a similar way. The form cancer takes will depend on the kind of cell tissue in which it originates and the nature of the body services it intrudes on. So cancers of the breast, liver, skin or bone marrow each take different forms as they grow. Their symptoms are different because the tissues in which they develop have different modes of behaviour.

To some extent this accounts for the mystery that has arisen about cancer. Some cancers, like most skin cancers, are easily treated because they are often quickly noticed, easily reached medically, and any contributing environmental factor, like over-suntanning, easily acted upon. Other cancers at similar stages of growth and in similar cell types, say, in the liver or the stomach, tend to remain unnoticed and unattended to, are difficult to reach medically and often by the time they are noticed are so advanced that little can be done. This complexity tends to puzzle people used to identifying illnesses with specific germs and specific effects and is the paradox of cancer. It is possible for people to have cancer without ever knowing it, to live to a robust old age, die of some other cause and have their cancer discovered only at post-mortem; others have easily-cured, painless cancer, and still others have rapidly-growing painful cancer to which they quickly succumb. It all depends where in the body it takes root. Cancer is not necessarily painful, nor does its mere presence spell death. Cancer kills by its action of spreading into vital organs; so long as a growth is not near a vital organ, life is preserved. Cancer causes pain only if it spreads across a pain receptor network. When cancer spreads and forms metastases in other parts of the body, these are often more serious because they are sited in vital and hard-to-reach organs like the brain or the liver.

WHAT CAUSES CANCER?

Obviously if we knew what caused cancer, there would be no mystery and we would probably be well on the way towards curing it. Our problems arise because we do not know precisely how cancer starts, nor at what point in the long chain of events involved in the life of cell tissue it occurs. Does something go wrong in the cell itself? Or perhaps in the systems that feed and drain the cell? Is it an inherited flaw? Or is it something in the environment — something we come into contact with that 'infects' us — something we eat, drink, or perhaps a bug, a virus, we catch?

Some of these questions we can answer with a degree of confidence. Take heredity for example. Many people worry that they can *inherit* a cancer-proneness if one or both of their parents had cancer. However, most experts believe that, by and large, cancer-proneness is not directly inherited except in a handful of rare instances; some people may inherit skin excessively sensitive to sunlight (*xeroderma pigmentosum*); others may inherit a condition whereby polyps (small protrusions) hang down in the colon and rectum and, through irritation, may become cancerous (*polyposis coli*). Neither *cause* cancer, but instead make the individual cancer-prone in that specific area. *Retinoblastoma*, a condition whereby a growth develops in the retina of young children, is probably the only truly inherited cancer and that is a very rare condition indeed.

Of the major cancers — breast, lung, bowel — the role played by any possible inherited factor is very low in comparison to environmental influences. If your mother had breast cancer, for example, you might inherit a greater risk of developing it as it does seem, to a mild extent, to run in families. Research though, has not been able to sort out whether this is due to direct genetic inheritance, or through being raised in a family where inter-personal, behavioural and dietary habits (judged more likely to cause you to develop cancer) are at work. Similarly, in lung cancer, smoking is such a powerful causative factor that even if you inherit a vulnerability but don't smoke, in all likelihood you'll never get cancer. If you do inherit a 'proneness', it is no more than that; you need something else — some carcinogenic influence from the environment perhaps — to actually trigger off an actual growth.

By far the most well-established 'causes' linked to cancer are known cancer-creating agents in nature. We call these *carcinogens* and can identify two basic kinds: those that are naturally-occurring and those that are man-made.

Naturally-occurring carcinogens are surprizingly common. The sun is one example. Specific kinds of light rays have been linked to skin and lip cancers and greater incidences of these cancers are reported in hot, sunny climates. Certain geo-graphical regions too, are known to have higher incidence rates for some cancers. In Switzerland, for example, thyroid cancers used to be common due to a lack of naturally-occurring iodine in some cantons. In Egypt a common kind of bladder cancer has been linked to the presence of a local parasite in rivers used for bathing. People living in tropical countries tend to have different kinds of cancer to those living in colder climates, partly due to differences in diet, food storage and preparation, and personal hygiene. Even fluctuations in soil conditions have been associ-ated with cancer. Parts of East Anglia in England, and certain regions in North Wales, have higher than average incidences of stomach cancer linked to the presence of greater concentrates of peat in the soil.

This is not to say that Switzerland, Egypt, the Tropics, North Wales or the fenlands are dangerous places to inhabit with carcinogens lying in wait for you round every corner. Far from it; where cancers have been linked to these factors, it is inevitably in the sense that individuals may be over-exposed to specific carcinogens which create the kind of chronic irritation that sets the scene for cancer. Chronic over-exposure to the sun works like that, and the Egyptian parasite mentioned above doesn't 'give' people cancer; it sets up a chronic inflammation of the lining of the bladder wall, which in time can become cancerous.

Man-made carcinogens are essentially naturally-occurring in the sense that they are present in nature, but through industrialization, mining, manufacturing and so on, human contact with them is intensified. We are all familiar with the links between cancer and working with asbestos or being exposed to radiation, but there are many others. Nickel, chrome and coal workers have been found to be at increased risk from cancer, as have hardwood workers, agricultural workers, workers in the dry cleaning and laundry industries, and others. Those working with alcohol, even bartenders, have been shown to be statistically more likely to get certain kinds of cancer than other people. Again, exposure to these man-made carcinogens does not in itself automatically cause cancer; it merely increases the risk.

This important point is one we will return to later. When we identify a carcinogen it means that the substance can set up an irritation which can become cancerous, but do not think of it as the actual 'cancer-causer'. Other factors modify the effects of a carcinogen. Some people exposed to carcinogens do not get cancer at all. Some carcinogens are carcinogenic for some species but not for others. Coal tar is carcinogenic for rabbits, for example, but has no effect on dogs or rats. And remember, statistics are general tendencies implying the possibility of links between carcinogens and cancer, not actual cause and effect. Statistics have to be interpreted very carefully. To give you one example, people who use drinking water from rivers in industrial regions, such as the Thames or the Mississippi, are statistically more prone to cancer than those drinking water from unpolluted rivers, but not everyone drinking water from the Thames in London has cancer or will inevitably get it.

The point is that the presence of carcinogens in the environment is only the first part of the chain that eventually ends in cancer. Industrialization certainly helps to increase risk, but it alone, along with the kind of geographical factors outlined earlier, play relatively minor roles in causing the most frequently occurring cancers. Social and cultural factors play by far the largest role in exposing individuals to carcinogens, and generally dictate what kinds of cancers predominate in any given society or community. So let's now examine the way social and cultural influences have shaped patterns of cancer incidence.

Social and cultural factors play a part in exposing an individual to carcinogens long before anything else. Smoking is a socially-approved habit that has little to do with working in an industry or living in a particular geographical region, and a growing child is much more likely to be exposed to tobacco smoke than any industrial or geographic carcinogen. Moreover, he or she is likely to be exposed to the effects of smoke from shortly after birth onwards. In fact, social and cultural factors are the major reasons why lung cancer has progressed from being a rare disease in 1900 to being the second biggest killer (after heart attacks) of men and women in the West today.

Consider the history of tobacco smoking. In primitive societies, leaves are dried, rolled and smoked. In this state, heavy smoking is difficult as the tobacco is too strong, so consumption is low and lung cancer rare. Much the same pattern occurred when tobacco was introduced into Britain and America. At first cigarettes were rough, smoking moderate and lung cancer rare. Late in the nineteenth century, though, manufacturers, eager to increase consumption of their products, grew and refined much lighter tobacco leaves making them easier to smoke. Consumption increased and so did lung cancer. But the real 'push' for cigarette consumption came in the First and Second World Wars when the US army in particular actively encouraged soldiers to smoke and distributed free cigarettes like sweets. Advertising and media images used in civilian life all added to the *socially approved* idea that cigarette smoking was both a fashionable and safe thing to do. After all, if governments, health authorities and the army approved, how was the ordinary person in the street to think otherwise? Cigarette consumption grew enormously after the Second World War and with it the incidence of lung cancer first in men then, more recently, in women.

Similar socio-cultural patterns can be identified in the incidence rates of other major cancers, stomach, breast and genital cancers. Stomach cancer, for example, has a particularly high incidence in Japan and other parts of the Far East where diets are high in salt and pickles. Food is also often eaten very hot and meal times, especially in traditional homes, are highly structured, formal affairs. These factors have all been linked to cancer; it is argued, for instance, that such diets, eaten in relatively unrelaxed circumstances, may routinely cause inflammation and discomfort and this, plus possible carcinogens in smoked, spiced, heavily salted, or pickled foods, does the damage.

Stomach cancer, although still a big killer in the West, is steadily declining in incidence due, it is believed, to the changing eating habits in our culture; people are taking more care with their diets, turning more to fresh and natural foods and away from preserved food. A fascinating example of the effects of cultural habits in this respect is provided by studies of what happens to Japanese people when they emigrate to Hawaii or California; the incidence of stomach cancer drops off and Japanese immigrants' cancer incidence patterns become more typical of their adopted countries. Lung cancer increases and, of particular significance, the incidence of breast cancer — rare in Japanese women — increases markedly.

Cultural values, of course, affect more than just smoking, eating and drinking habits. They also affect how we relate to each other, how we live and how we plan our families. There is some evidence to believe that the increased incidence of breast cancer in Western societies is due in part to women bearing fewer children. Cultures which encourage families to have more pregnancies have lower breast cancer rates than others. Pregnancy with its hormonal changes, is believed to provide some protection against cancer in women. Lots of fats and sugars in the diet have also been linked to breast cancer risk. Again, cultural factors influence what people like to eat and we are all familiar with the effect of advertising on dietary habits.

Cervical cancer offers a particularly illuminating example of just how cultural factors work and how powerful they can be. This is the one kind of cancer in which medical research and medical screening measures have changed the face of the disease's progress. Not only are very effective treatments available which ensure almost complete recovery if it is spotted early enough, but the Pap smear test has become so widely accepted by gynaecologists and their patients, that most cases are spotted at the check-ups many women willingly undergo. It is a painless, efficient and culturally-approved preventive measure — a triumph of medical research and public relations.

With early detection and efficient treatment, cervical cancer no longer kills women as it used to. However, it remains a serious problem because prompt diagnosis has had no effect on the *incidence* of cervical cancer; more women in the West are getting this form of cancer than ever before. Analyses of social trends over the past fifty years have clearly linked the increase to changes in cultural habits and values, in particular to changes in sexual morality. Looser attitudes towards making love, crises like the two world wars in which freer, more temporary relationships became socially tolerated, and particularly the permissiveness of the 1960s and 1970s, all mean that people make love more often, start younger and have more partners; the result increases an individual's chances of being exposed to sexually-transmitted disease. The increase in cervical cancer, herpes, AIDS, the increase in common venereal diseases (like syphilis and gonorrhoea) are all part of this syndrome. Less public attention has been drawn to the male side of this picture, but it parallels the pattern of cervical cancer; cancer of the testicles is today the most frequent cancer found in men under the age of thirty-five.

The point to realize, in an attempt to understand cancer, is that these two key elements — the presence of carcinogens and behaviour that exposes individuals to them — constitute the first two links in the causal chain. Cancer is a natural phenomenon, but carcinogens do their damage only if repeated and frequent exposure to them takes place. This inevitably occurs when patterns of exposure become well-established as social habits. But is this enough? Can we stop our examination there, blame industrialization, tobacco companies, loose morals, junk food, or the fashion for suntans for causing cancer and leave it at that? Obviously not. We are all exposed to cultural pressures, we all routinely come into contact with carcinogens, but not all of us get cancer. Not all smokers get lung cancer. Not all people eating the same diet get stomach cancer. Not every permissive lover gets genital cancer.

To complete the chain and to find the vital missing link that makes sense of everything discussed so far we must turn to the third and final part of the cancer chain; what goes on inside the body.

The most important element in the cancer chain obviously takes place within the body itself. Carcinogens in the environment carry the cancer-causing potential, but what is it that happens in the body for a cancerous growth to start?

Whatever form the carcinogen in contact with the body takes, be it a chemical, nicotine in tobacco smoke, a virus or harmful radiation, its primary action appears to be to damage the cells in the area of immediate contact. Think of this as occurring in a straightforward way, like sunburn. Over-exposure destroys cells and they have to be replaced. Constant over-exposure, though, does more than just damage cells; it changes their ability to produce accurate reproductions of themselves. Instead, immature and imperfect cells are produced which are not entirely suited to their job, and not able to cope as well as normal cells.

In a very simple sense this is all carcinogens coming into contact with the body do. This is believed to be a fairly routine occurrence for practically all of us over-exposed to a carcinogen for periods of time. If exposure to the carcinogen ceases, these immature cells die off, are overwhelmed by normal cells and the target area returns to its former healthy self. This is what we mean when we talk of cancer being a part of living and probably accounts for the benign growths or cell-changes many of us contract from time to time.

Something else has to happen for this initial damage to become cancerous. What is described above is termed a pre-cancerous state, purely a precondition for any possible development of cancer. For a damaged cell area to become cancerous, the body's internal support systems have to fail to deal properly with the existence of this pre-cancerous condition. How can this happen? To answer this, let's look at how the body protects itself from disease in general.

THE BODY'S SUPPORT SYSTEMS

Many people are inclined to think of illness in a slightly old-fashioned way. Diseases are caused by germs that get into the body and if powerful enough, they inflict great damage. In a sense this is quite true; some infections, like smallpox, malaria, polio and influenza work in exactly this manner, and we deal with them by trying to prevent their entry into the body. However, with diseases like cancer, we have to modify this view of illness, appreciating instead that the body survives for the most part by a quite intricate interdependency with so-called 'germs'. In fact, the body uses 'germs' in various ways to stay alive. Bacteria in the intestines help manage the body's wastes. The body is not a totally stable, sterile environment. Its own actions, fluctuations, inconsistencies and weaknesses can create some of the circumstances in which diseases thrive. Above all, the body's self-defence systems can fluctuate quite markedly from time to time and in quite surprising ways.

The body's defensive network, the immune system, is one of three key support or servicing systems in the body which together more or less control how the body behaves at any given moment. The body's cells, the vital organs, bones and muscular system are the basics which give structure and form to the body, but it is the body's support systems that organize what actually goes on inside.

The *central nervous system* is the body's basic communications network, linking the highest centres of the mind (or brain) with the lowest — the tip of our toes. It is spread throughout the body, comprising thousands of nerves relaying information and commands continuously back and forth. Our muscles are controlled by nervous impulses, all our senses feed input to the brain through the nervous system, and just about everything we do — right down to how fast the heart beats — gets done through the agencies of the central nervous system (CNS). The CNS provides a fast, minute-by-minute picture of what's happening in our bodies and in the world outside. How we think, feel, see, how we act or react, is determined by the information received in the higher nervous centres of this system. Above all, our consciousness resides in the CNS.

The nervous system could be termed the body's central 'living' or 'coping' system. If someone stands on your foot, it is the CNS that tells you about it and the CNS that moves your hands to push the offender away. If you have to solve a difficult moral dilemma, it's the same CNS that will keep you lying awake all night doing so. In short, it is the CNS that is most vulnerable to stress and which can override, to some extent, the activity of the other systems. It's through the CNS, for example, that the heart is kept overactive and blood pressure high, in people who can't relax; business executives, for instance, who keep adrenalin flowing through their systems when there is no physical reason for doing so. It's also the CNS that keeps parts of the body in states of chronic stress; making you, for example, chronically tense, chronically depressed, or even chronically over-active. Headaches, insomnia, constipation, backache and a whole range of other common complaints often originate in disturbances in CNS functioning. The CNS, in sum, monitors our psychological states and provides the physiological match or parallel that goes with them. If you're sitting down relaxed and you suddenly remember something you've forgotten to do, it's your CNS that sends the shivers of anxiety through your body, and alerts all the other systems in unison.

The endocrine or hormonal system works very closely with the nervous system and starts high up in the brain in the pituitary gland and the hypothalamus. The hormone system operates via key centres which control and regulate the activity of cells all over the body. Acting through chemical messengers in the blood, hormonal secretions instruct cells to reproduce, or not, and dictate the pace at which they do so. The hormonal system is the body's balancing network, regulating and stabilizing the internal environment. It is also responsible for mental and physical efficiency, for maintaining proper sleep/wake patterns, proper growth, and energy levels. It's the hormonal system, for instance, that dictates how quickly we digest food and burn up energy and, of course, to relate it to the activity of cancer cells, how well supplied in protein these cells are kept, and how fast or slowly damaged cells reproduce themselves.

The immune system is the support system most closely involved with the protection of cells where cancers may grow. It operates largely through its own lymph network which drains each cell area and destroys any unwanted bacteria; but immune agents also circulate in the blood supply protecting organs and the blood flow to cell areas.

The important thing about these three support systems is that they work very much as a team, interacting with one another to service cells and body organs, while still functioning as components of one cohesive system. The immune system operates rather like a naval task force with a mixture of different ships working together as a team. When a smaller immune unit meets an alien entity it might be able to deal with it itself, but if not, it sends out messengers and larger or more powerful units pitch in to help out. So closely integrated is this system that some clusters of killer units only operate in a set sequence to destroy foreign cells; each on its own has a negligible influence, but acting together they achieve the necessary effect. By the same token, each acting in the wrong sequence renders the effects harmless. Teamwork and co-ordination are what matter.

The hormonal systems work in a similar way; control and balance in the body being achieved by sets of opposing hormonal agents acting on one another. Getting the balance right means knowing how much of one must be secreted to balance the other. Teamwork. Most of us, too, are familiar with the way the central nervous system is responsible for both alerting and arousing the body through the sympathetic nervous network and relaxing it through the para-sympathetic system. Balance and co-ordination between the two are essential for the efficiency and healthy operation of the body.

Surprisingly, these three body systems are very vulnerable

to quite commonplace influences. Anxiety, for example, especially if it's highly specific and chronic, can change the level and efficiency with which the nervous system functions; intense or chronic emotions can interfere with the normal regulatory activity of the endocrine system through reducing the degree and balance of secretion of a wide range of hormones. But most important, commonplace events can interfere with the efficiency of the immune system.

Research has shown the immune system's vulnerability at quite ordinary levels. Losing sleep, for example, for whatever reason, or having irregular disturbed sleep can reduce the levels of functioning of certain aspects of the immune system. The immune system also fluctuates quite extensively during the course of the day; early in the morning, for instance, your system is probably at its best, slowly losing its efficiency as the day passes. Eating a meal, running to catch a train, coping with traffic, having a drink, having an argument, all have their effects on the immune system.

Being overweight affects your immune system. People with excess weight are more inclined to die from infectious diseases than those without — quite apart from the other known risks, such as heart disease, diabetes and gallstones, that obese people face. Some studies have shown that fluctuations in protein cause fluctuations in the efficiency of the immune system.

Last, but by no means least, *stress* has been reliably demonstrated to have a wide range of effects on immune functioning. Early work on tuberculosis (TB) victims, for example, showed that upset and distress due to such crises as change of job, divorce, or money worries, were fairly clearly linked to an occurrence of TB. Other, more recent, research has established links between the experience of psychological stress and upper respiratory tract infections (cold, flu, coughs), recovery from mononucleosis (glandular fever), herpes simplex, ulcerative gingivitis (trench mouth) and cancer, to name but some.

THE THREE STEPS TO CANCER

What has this got to do with the cancer process? A good deal, because it completes, as it were, our discussion of the cancer chain. Now it is clear that getting cancer involves not just carcinogens, but a rather more complex set of circumstances.

First, we require the presence of a carcinogen or several carcinogens together. We need irritation, injury, inflammation — something that disturbs or damages cells in a specific area. This irritation can come from any of several sources; in our food, in the smoke or air we inhale, in exposure to radiation, sunshine, or whatever. In any event, we require that the irritation activates the body's cell- or tissue-repair function. Cancer rarely occurs spontaneously without some form of actual invasion or irritation. Its very nature resides in the fact that it is a normal body-repair and regeneration function gone wrong. Let's call this *Step 1.*

Secondly, we require that within the body, the individual's normal tendency to remove him or herself from a source of irritation does not take place. Through conscious (central nervous system) choices or overriding emotional (endocrine) reactions, the pain and discomfort messages sent from the damaged site are ignored or, if reacted to, side-tracked or weakened by poor nervous and endocrine system teamwork. The result is that the damaged cells have to cope with exposure to carcinogens as best they can — thus producing flawed and immature new cells. This is *Step 2.* Not yet cancer, but ready and waiting to become malignant.

Once established, we require, finally, for the new mass to turn cancerous, the body's immune system to fail to react adequately to its presence. Again, it very much looks as though the activity of the nervous and endocrine systems confuses the local immune reaction, and the immune cells that would ordinarily identify the new mass as immature cells and destroy them, instead treat the new growth as a valid part of the local system. Whether this occurs because the immune system actually does accept the neoplasm, or because it is too weak or vulnerable to destroy the cells is unclear. Given the fact that the immune system does accept some benign growths without destroying them, and accepts some for a time (like warts) and destroys them later, it seems that both mechanisms are at work. Either way, this is *Step 3*.

The three steps share one common denominator — whether they occur or not is dictated very largely by the way individuals behave and the responses they make to environmental and social pressures. It is, remember, a matter of individual choice that most carcinogens are brought into the body in the first place. We choose to smoke too much, we choose to eat unhealthy substances, to drink excessively, to sunbathe to a cinder, and so on. People also choose to neglect the proper care of their bodies and it is this that mostly accounts for the vulnerabilities of functions in the efficiency of the immune and endocrine systems. Lastly, remember that conscious choice (enacted through the central nervous system) is by far the most powerful force at work in the body. It alone is capable of overriding, confusing and deregulating the delicately balanced activity of the immune and endocrine systems.

To go any further in looking for a pattern of somatopsychic functioning that causes cancer, we must look very closely at how the individual who *chooses* to expose himself or herself to a carcinogen and who *chooses* to override body-protection functions works. We must now look at cancer and the mind to see what light is thrown on this investigation by studies on people who get cancer. Afterwards we will return in Chapter 3 to put the pieces together and elucidate the links between how we behave and how cancer starts.

CHAPTER 2
Cancer and Personality

If we accept that the way an individual behaves in life can predispose him or her to getting cancer, then we need to know something about what these patterns of behaviour are. Can we identify 'types' of people or personalities that are more prone to getting cancer than others? This question has intrigued doctors since Ancient Greek times and many attempts have been made to answer it, most of them presuming some kind of link between emotional upset and the onset of cancer.

It was once thought that people who were habitually gloomy, or experienced massive grief or misery, were vulnerable to cancer. Earlier this century, when psychiatric research became a little more scientific, terms like 'depressive', 'inward-turning' and 'over-sensitive' began to be applied to cancer sufferers. They were also called 'self-pitying' and, above all, 'repressive', tending to keep feelings of anger and jealousy under tight control. This idea of the cancer-prone person having a 'repressive' personality attained great prominence amongst Freudian theorists, who described cancer victims as repressing their emotions so harshly that normal body and psychological development could not take place.

30

While these early ideas about the cancer-prone personality were interesting, they remained too general to be of much use to doctors trying to understand the links between the mind and what was known about cancer growths. Research into other illnesses usually turned up very similar findings; TB sufferers and asthmatics, for example, were described in very similar ways. This made it hard to know whether the descriptions resulted from illness or pointed to a basic, predisposing factor in personality. Most people naturally become grief-stricken, depressed and repressed if told they have cancer; further, many ill people in hospital display similar personality traits.

After 1950, better research methods resulted in more closely-defined studies. Five kinds of research have now been conducted on cancer victims. *Retrospective* studies where cancer victims are researched and their past lives examined for clues once the diagnosis is known. These studies ask the question, 'what were these people like before they got cancer?' *Prospective* studies ask a similar question, but do it the other way round; groups of people are investigated at an early stage in their lives and then followed up later to see what kinds of early factors could be linked to the development of cancer. *Contiguous* studies look at how cancer victims cope once they have cancer and ask the question, 'Do some kinds of personalities survive longer or better than others?' *Animal* studies examine cancer in laboratory animals and look at all these issues, but in more tightly controlled ways. Lastly, some research on how *unorthodox medical practitioners* achieve their effects has contributed to our knowledge about the role of the mind in cancer survival.

Retrospective studies　　These have mostly supported the earlier ideas about depressed or repressive personality patterns being associated with cancer, but have done so more objectively and in more detail.

In Scotland, for example, a team of researchers examined lung cancer victims, using questionnaires to measure personality and childhood behaviour (Kissen, 1963). This, one of the better studies of the time since it compared cancer victims with other hospital patients, i.e. people in similar circumstances, helped Kissen establish the fact that the early lives of cancer subjects differed from those of subjects with other diseases. He found cancer sufferers frequently had a limited ability to express their emotions both as children and as they grew older. Later studies by the same team confirmed this finding and other work on other kinds of cancer established much the same pattern.

In a different study, conducted in America, a research team gave a personality test to women after they had had a negative Pap test (cervical smear), but before a diagnosis of cancer was confirmed. Later, when the diagnoses were confirmed, the personality tests on those without cancer were compared to those with cancer. When the smear test results were later given, the personality tests on those with cancer were compared to those without. Cancer victims were found to express more 'hopeless' feelings that those without cancer, but also to have suffered recent emotional loss — a long-term relationship had ended or changed for the worse.

One other study was of considerable interest. Le Shan and his associates in America studied cancer victims using a variety of methods including questionnaires, psychotherapy and projective tests; they found that the childhood experiences of most cancer patients were characterized by a lack of (or subdued) emotional response and a kind of stoic and bland acceptance of normal ups and downs. Le Shan noted, too, that as adults his patients felt isolated and often powerless in the world. Significantly again many cancer patients had lost key relationships prior to the onset of cancer. In typical cases he wrote, '[for these people] ... intense interpersonal relationships appear difficult and dangerous. When a strong, meaningful relationship was found ... this became the centre of the individual's life ... He functioned adequately but superficially in other life areas. [When this relationship was lost] Attempts to find substitute relationships failed, and the patient underwent a period of intense despair which was later repressed. Within a period of six months to eight years after the loss ... the first signs of malignancy were noted.' (Le Shan, 1959, p. 12)

Other research teams have examined cancer victims using this retrospective method of study, but with different tools and, in some cases, different findings. One series of studies in London studied women with breast cancer and found that losing a 'loved one', being depressed, extroverted or introverted bore no relationship to having breast cancer. What did, though, were measures of anger suppression and anxiety expression; breast cancer victims tended to restrain their anger more than other women and to express less anxiety.

Retrospective studies have reinforced the idea that cancer victims hold their feelings in too much and helped us to see that this, coupled with a feeling of helplessness and hopelessness, seems to be the mark of general cancer-proneness. However, interpretation of the studies has to be cautious because of the enormous complexity of both the human personality and the different effects various kinds of cancer have. In one study anger and anxiety suppression was found to be an important factor in women under fifty, but not for those over fifty. While this does not invalidate the original finding it suggests the need for rigorous analysis of terms like 'anger suppression'. Let's look at other areas of research first before trying to place these findings in context. Remember, at this level, what is important is an accurate overall picture of the role played by personality in the development of cancer, not simply to focus on 'anger' or 'anxiety' in isolation.

Contiguous studies   What happens to people once they have cancer? This is a somewhat easier problem to investigate than others and considerable evidence now shows that psychological factors are significantly involved in how long people survive after cancer is discovered.

The basic design of the research is quite straightforward: cancer sufferers with the same kind of cancer, at the same stage, are examined and tested once a cancer diagnosis has been made; then, after some time, the results are re-examined to see if any personality or psychological factor can be related to such things as length of survival, the speed with which tumours grow, and so on. Here you are comparing as it were, cancer victims with other cancer victims, long-term survivors versus short-term survivors.

Consistent findings, using this approach, have been reported by a variety of research teams in a variety of countries. One team in the United States found that long-term survivors often enjoyed closer personal relationships than short-term survivors; they also seemed less emotionally distressed and took a more active and interested part in their treatment, trying to help the hospital help them in the sense of appreciating how vital their own co-operation was to their survival. Short-term survivors often resigned themselves to the inevitable and were inclined to give up and feel hopeless almost immediately.

Researchers at King's College Hospital in London have made a major contribution to our knowledge in this area. In well-controlled studies of women with breast cancer, it was found that those who survived longer displayed a determined 'fighting spirit'; this was often combined with a fortuitous denial of reality in which the shock of having the disease was somehow kept at bay and prevented from overwhelming the patient and making her feel hopeless.

Poor survivors, in contrast, showed either a stoic, fatalistic reaction or a deep sense of hopelessness and helplessness. The same team reported that patients who adjusted poorly to mastectomy (the breast removal operation) were more neurotic and depressive than those who adjusted well.

In essence, then, psychological factors do appear to play a significant role in surviving cancer; the more determined you are to fight for your life, the stronger your will to live, the more likely you are to live. Being able to translate this power into effective emotional and practical outlets further guarantees your safety. More about this in later chapters.

Prospective studies   These studies are by far the most time-consuming and expensive, but they are undoubtedly the most useful. Very simply, the investigation is begun on a number of normal, healthy people, usually when they are young adults. They are given a range of psychological tests, are medically examined, their habits and backgrounds noted and so on. Then, as these people age, test results of those who get cancer are compared with those who don't, or with those who get other diseases. Also test material of those who survive cancer longer or better can be examined and a picture of the individual's psychological functioning long beforehand built up. Of course, all this takes a long time. A shorter way, which some research teams have taken, is to go back and study groups of people who for one reason or another all once underwent psychological tests and then look at the results for cancer victims. One such study, begun in 1977, is engaged in looking at the records of over 50,000 students from the Universities of Harvard and Pennsylvania in the United States. Another team went back over the MMPI records (a personality test) of patients entering a Kansas veterans hospital over the years and compared test results for cancer versus non-cancer patients.

A number of prospective studies have now been conducted in various parts of the world, from Berkeley in California to Sweden and even Yugoslavia. Not all have used as large numbers as the Harvard study, but they have all contributed to the growing evidence that psychological factors play a significant role in the development of cancer.

In the Yugoslav investigation, starting in 1965, 1,353 elderly people in the small village of Crvenka were examined in great detail, medically, psychologically and sociologically, and then re-examined periodically. In 1976, all causes of deaths of people in the sample were noted and then the data examined to see which factors could be linked to cancer death. Interestingly enough, smoking and immunological measures were also taken in this study and they permit, in part, an assessment of the relative importance of psychological, immunological and behavioural factors acting together. Overall, the authors found that psychological factors such as the repression of emotions (defined as a proneness to being 'anti-emotional') and above all, a general spirit of hopelessness, were the most reliable predictors of cancer death, more so than physical measures, such as blood cholesterol and lymphocite levels.

Those who were able to express anger openly significantly decreased their likelihood of getting cancer, and when feeling anger and feeling 'hopeless' scores were compared for those who died from cancer and from circulatory disease, it was found that those people who got cancer inevitably scored highly on hopelessness, while those getting circulatory disease scored highly on anger.

Interesting findings also emerged from the point of view of the physiological measures employed. Under stress, i.e. when upset for one reason or another, cancer people showed marked fluctuations in their blood cholesterol levels with a physiological struggle seeming to go on within the individual as he or she tried to minimize the upset. (High cholesterol levels are associated with stress.) When compared to non-cancer people and to those with heart disease, a characteristic cancer pattern emerged; while heart or stroke disease sufferers showed higher levels of cholesterol than cancer sufferers, cancer victims tended to show consistently more fluctuations of their levels under stress. In short, cancer victims, while appearing 'unemotional' to the onlooker, were under considerable and volatile stress inside. Interestingly enough, lymphocite levels (a measure of immune function) were also lower in cancer people than in others, suggesting to the researchers a chronic lowering of immune function. Lastly, smoking in these people was studied and found to be an important predictor of lung cancer, but not as important a predictor as psychological variables.

Here we have confirmatory evidence of the role of psychological factors in cancer from as far away (culturally and geographically) as Yugoslavia. Closer to home, the evidence is very similar. In the Kansas study, for example, it was found that cancer victims had earlier shown a well established personality pattern characterized as being prone to despair, being repressed and trying not to express emotions of distress (defined as a denial of hysteria). Again, the idea of someone struggling not to show what was going on inside emerges – again, this time, it was shown to be a distinct personality trait before the individual developed cancer. One of the authors of the Harvard-Pennsylvania study I mentioned earlier suggested that the failure to express emotions in a straightforward manner put greater pressure on other means of expressing stress like smoking or drinking. They found in one study that, while other psychological variables were not important in predicting Hodgkins' Disease (a form of cancer), those who smoked heavily, drank coffee to excess or had become overweight as young adults before developing the disease were more likely to get the disease than those who did not.

By far the most important prospective study to date has been the one conducted at John Hopkins University, Baltimore, in America. Dr C.B. Thomas and her team of investigators set out after the Second World War to study medical students at the university; they took part in a wide range of tests, background questionnaires and so on as they came to university and have been followed up annually ever since.

Thomas and her colleagues have put together a list of characteristics, measured when young adults, of those doctors who later contracted or died of cancer and which distinguish them from doctors suffering from other diseases. Let's examine each in turn.

Early family life of cancer people   Perhaps the most significant of the study's findings was that cancer people did not feel as close to their parents as did other people, and those subjects who later developed heart conditions. Cancer people inevitably reported a lack of contact or lack of warmth between themselves and their parents. Significantly, this feeling was more marked in those who later developed a more serious form of cancer than in those who had milder forms (like skin cancer) or benign tumours. And, remember, these were feelings reported by the individuals when as young adults they had only just left home; we can be fairly certain they reflected pretty accurately how they felt about their parents. Very often they could not put their finger on actual instances of trauma or distress, just a general feeling of distance. Of considerable importance, too, was the finding that the cancer group's responses were most like those of subjects who later developed mental problems, or those who committed suicide. That is, those who later had trouble coping with life had also reported feeling distant to their parents in their youth. Unlike the future cancer victims, however, people who later developed heart problems reported that they felt closer to their parents.

Evidence of nervous tension   In confirmation of the above, Thomas also found cancer people to have displayed nervous habits as young adults that showed a degree of personal insecurity. When upset or under pressure, cancer people reported that they became obsessional, constantly checking and re-checking for imaginary lapses or omissions. The general tendency of cancer people was to express upset, not by saying so

or feeling distressed, but by getting fatigued; they often
complained of feeling too tired to do things, felt easily exhausted
and frequently felt depressed. Further, they also reported
wanting to eat or to smoke or drink as a means of allaying
nervous tension.

General interests and attitudes to life   At university, subjects
who later developed cancer were already showing an approach to
life that reflected their wariness about close personal relationships and about emotions. They tended for instance to shun
emotionally-stimulating activities like art, going to concerts, or
reading; Thomas comments that they seemed to be negative,
lacked spontaneity, and had little stamina for the vigour of full
living. Rorschach and other in-depth studies showed that this
component of avoidance was a feature of cancer people's records
when compared to other illness groups. Again an ambivalence in
personality functioning emerged in these tests, especially in the
area of relationships; cancer people were unsure of their feelings
and seemed to swing between intensely positive or negative
feelings without the balance necessary for proper relationships.
These findings suggest that cancer people demonstrated
ignorance early on of how to relate to other people emotionally.
Because of their insecurity and distance from their parents, they
seemed to lack the freedom to explore and express intense
feelings in the protection of a safe relationship. This fact may
well be closely linked to the earlier findings of Le Shan and
others, that many cancer people seem to go through life experiencing one very intense close relationship and then, when it goes
or is lost, never recovering to form another one. More of all this
later. Note, incidentally, that the in-depth tests showed the
same internal state to be present in cancer people as the
Yugoslav studies did.

Animal studies   As you can imagine, the problems of
doing research on animals are very different from those encoun-
tered in doing human research. For one thing, you can arrange
matters much more to your convenience; you can control just
about everything more reliably and monitor what happens very
much more carefully. In that sense, the animal findings on

cancer research have assumed very great prominence over the years, nowhere more so than on research linking stress to cancer.

One basic method in stress research though there are many different ways has been to take a strain of, say, mice, which have been bred very carefully so as not to be either 'inbred', or too different from each other in terms of their life experiences, exposure to infections and so on. Then, two groups from the same breeding strain (and therefore to all purposes identical) would be given cancer (usually by transplanting identical tumours into identical sites), and then separated into two sets of living conditions, again identical in every aspect but with one crucial difference between the two groups — one would be exposed to stress and the other not. Careful note would then be made of the rate of tumour growth and length of survival time before death.

A number of consistent findings have emerged from studies run like this. Suffice to say that animal research overall has not only demonstrated the importance of the link between stress and cancer, but has also confirmed the general direction of much of the psychological research mentioned elsewhere in this chapter. Animal studies in the future may even tell us a great deal more; already there is evidence that stress factors also have an effect on the development of metastases in animals and it may be possible to prevent cancer in animals who have been given cancer artificially by arranging their environment so that they can cope with it better.

Unorthodox or alternative forms of medicine
Alternative medicine encompasses a very broad spectrum of theories, ranging from holistic approaches stressing lifestyle, diet, natural cures and the like, to faith healers and spiritualists. Most adhere very strongly to the notion that if you decide to do something about your problems and you are correctly motivated, then the effect of belief, faith or natural remedy will ensure that your body is better equipped to fight the illness. They are helped in this argument by the considerable evidence in *orthodox* medical literature for what is regarded as the spontaneous remission of cancer; that is, the number of cases where recovery occurs for no known medical reason or intervention.

Without going into these alternative approaches in detail let me say that the problem is that all too often we only have the word of the practitioner, or the word of his or her patients to go on. Like the earlier Freudian case reports, these can be very interesting and generate useful hypotheses, but active research and clear formulations are required to substantiate these claims. Very few alternative practitioners have either carried out proper research, or indeed even reported their theories in a clear and researchable way. A fair proportion of alternative theorists use ideas and constructs that are, with the best will in the world, hard to relate to psychology in general, let alone the kind of mind-body issues spotlighted in this book. Undeniably, some practitioners make very real contact with their patients, and offer genuine help. I would, however, not always subscribe to *their* interpretations of what they do. Indeed, like many other orthodox practitioners, I tend to be wary of what I can't understand or see and I definitely draw the line at interpretations that incorporate extra-terrestrial or supernatural effects.

However, there are a number of practitioners who work outside orthodox medicine, but who nevertheless have provided acceptable information, research reports or hypotheses: I have confined my investigations to those.

Probably the most important reports have emerged from the clinic of O. Carl and Stephanie Simonton in Fort Worth, Texas. Beginning in the late 1960s, this team explored a range of psychological approaches in an attempt to uncover techniques that might help patients build up their psychological resistance to cancer. Encounter groups, meditation, positive thinking, group therapy, biofeedback, mind dynamics and others were examined, and eventually a programme was developed which seemed to help people fight cancer. Reports published by the authors suggested, in fact, that it was possible to teach people to use relaxation, imagery techniques and other behaviours to decrease their distress or tension and so help reduce tumour growth.

Other clinicians have reported similar effects. An Australian doctor, Christopher Magarey, has written about 'hostilic cancer therapy', arguing that the successes reported in alternative cancer clinics is often attributable, not to 'idiosyncratic

remedies', such as coffee enemas, liver juice, general immuniza-
tion, elimination of toxins, use of mistletoe, or laetrile, but rather
to 'one striking feature ... present in each clinic; the personal
charisma and profound spiritual (not necessarily religious) conviction of the medical director' (Magarey, 1983, p. 182). He ref-
ers for proof to a study on what actually happened when
charismatic healers worked with their clients, showing that the
key factor is the way the practitioner is able to make a patient
feel safe and at one with him or her. The same pattern has been
reported in studies of the effects of deep meditation and may
well occur at other clinics where the intense bond often noted
between doctor and patient helps the patient to become calm.
There is evidence that this calming influence affects the
patient's physiological functioning as well; heartbeat slows,
brainwaves relax and the autonomous nervous system relaxes.

Much the same can be said of the relationship between
hypnotist and client. Although hypnotism has long been
regarded as fringe medicine, it has become recognized in recent
years as a useful method of helping people adjust to problems.
Again, its greatest value seems to lie in the power the therapist
has to overcome the client's feeling of isolation; where a subject
is likely to be open to suggestion, the effects seem to be greater.
Hypnotists who work with cancer victims have remarked on how
cancer people are notably more open to suggestion than others.

What can we make of this? Quite apart from the 'ideology'
employed by various practitioners, what seems to be happening
is that they are fulfilling the deep psychological needs of their
cancer patients. Significantly, cancer victims turn to alternative
medicine usually after they have given up normal medicine, or
been given up by it. They are, of course, frightened and in need
of close personal support. Almost unwittingly perhaps, alternative medicine is attending to the psychological needs of cancer
patients that large numbers of orthodox practitioners have, in
the past, ignored or minimized. They are, in effect, putting into
practice much of what we have been discussing in this chapter.

SUMMING UP

Putting all these findings together, let me try to give you a picture of the personality and background characteristics likely to predispose an individual to cancer.

Childhood   Evidence seems to point to the fact that as the cancer-prone person grows up, he or she is exposed to a set of ideas and directives about how to behave, think and feel that involve a high degree of control; loose behaviour, childish attitudes, hysteria, distressing emotions and ordinary needy behaviours appear to be discouraged very early on in the child's life. Emotional expression seems then to be allowed or approved of in a very narrow, constricted way, in which being calm and 'adult' takes precedence over other forms. It seems that this pattern is developed and cemented by a very specific parent-child relationship in which the child is kept very close to the parent and not allowed much room to grow as an independent entity. Loss of, or serious change, in this relationship seems to leave the child powerless and unable to form an adequate substitute. If this change takes place at particularly vulnerable stages of the child's physical growth, he or she may be at risk to such childhood and adolescent cancers as leukaemia, lymphoma and Hodgkins' Disease.

Adolescence   Research findings of a lack of closeness and warmth between the cancer-prone individual and his or her parents, together with the evidence of cancer following on loss of a close, intimate relationship, suggest that the pattern of parent-child intimacy is disturbed in some way. A strong symbiotic relationship as a child seems to be followed in adolescence by a cooling or distancing relationship whereby the teenager feels increasingly ignored or pushed away in certain key respects. This need not be related to an actual 'loss' in the physical sense of, say, death of a parent (the evidence for loss or *specific* trauma is unsatisfactory), but appears to occur rather as a structured, long-term pattern of relationship in which the growing person's emotional needs are routinely neglected or ignored. This suggests that the child learns to disregard or ignore these same key parts of him or herself in line with this training and to adopt a disaffected view of important body and emotional needs.

Research suggests also that the parent-child relationship in cancer people was one-sided; the child was taught to focus on its parents' views and behaviours and to minimize his or her own view, own growth and own self-centredness. Very early on the cancer-prone child learns to feel relatively unimportant or powerless; there is little sense of having an important role to play as an individual (as opposed to a 'helper') in the family. The child is reared to perform parent-defined tasks, to accept them without question, to minimize his or her own view of reality and to deny or repress expressions of discord. We can hypothesize that a learned 'helplessness' develops early, and a strong dependency on an authority figure forms. The child can only think or behave in set ways; when these are lacking or confusing, the child has no resources for coping, other than to feel helpless, fatigued or depressed.

Adult life   Once the child grows up and leaves the immediate confines of family life, problems appear to arise in forming close bonds with others. Providing the individual can find someone similar to the dominant parent all may appear well, but this simply appears to maintain the status quo. The cancer-prone person is unable to cope with deep emotions and deep body needs and actually avoids them and/or their expression, both within him or herself and in others. He or she is also not well able to cope with life's normal stresses and tensions. Any relationship that *does not* require attention or action at these levels will support the family pattern. More demanding relationships will disturb and upset the individual, depending on the degree and severity of upset and the support given by the basic relationship.

Overall, cancer-prone individuals are vulnerable as adults to *stress* that threatens this underlying psychological pattern. Thus, divorce, death of a spouse, or other trauma can expose the underlying vulnerability, as too can the growing-up of one's own children; a healthy teenage son or daughter, for example, who challenges or threatens the mother's or father's psychological and emotional structure, may be abnormally threatening.

Cancer-prone people tend not to express emotions and this creates problems in forming coping habits. Day-to-day stresses and upsets become *too* big, too upsetting; the cancer-prone person, crippled by not being able to express upset and a feeling of helplessness and powerlessness, has to live with a routinely fluctuating level of internal body distress. All create both inter-personal problems and intra-psychic difficulties, not helped by the cancer person's characteristic and well-documented coping patterns — a kind of pretence that all is well, the use of obsessive-compulsive habits and the fatigue, lethargy and lack of energy created by feelings of helplessness.

The key component in this picture is the fact that through being reared in this rather emotionally sterile way, cancer-prone people often treat their own bodies with less care than other people do. In particular, they are more likely to ignore early signs of body stress or discomfort, are more likely to bottle things up inside and use 'passive' means of coping with upset (like eating or smoking) and lastly, are more likely to maintain their bodies' immune efficiency at a low level. All these effects become well-established habits that eventually alter the pattern of activity of the body's supportive systems — the central nervous, hormonal and immune systems. In Chapter 3, I will explore how these bad habits are linked to tumour growth.

CHAPTER 3
A New Psychology of Cancer

Now the findings reported in the last chapter must be placed in a coherent framework that will also accommodate the ideas developed earlier about body-mind interaction in the organism.

DEFINING THE PROBLEMS

In Chapter 1 I described research that suggested three basic steps were required for cancer actually to happen. *Step 1* specified that a carcinogen must be present in some form or another; *Step 2* required the failure of the body's central nervous and endocrine systems to either recognize or act on the damage done by the carcinogen present in step one: and finally, *Step 3* postulated that the body's immune system failed, probably through a lack of teamwork co-ordination, to attack and destroy the neoplasm, allowing it instead to become a part of its own system.

Adding detail to these three steps, some interesting facts

begin to emerge. Take *step 1*. The most common carcinogens
mentioned in cancer research in Westernized societies are the
following: *nicotine* in tobacco smoke, associated with lung
cancer, bladder cancer and liver cancer; *foodstuffs* associated
with breast cancer (sugar) and colorectal cancer (over-refined
food); *alcohol* associated with liver and throat cancer; *sexual
habits* associated with cervical and penile cancer; *radiation*
associated with skin cancer (over-exposure to sunshine). It is
important to realize that the chances of being over-exposed to
these everyday carcinogens are far greater than danger from
radiation from an atomic plant, say, or the radiation in granite
rocks around somewhere like Glasgow. Moreover, these everyday carcinogens are the ones to which we are exposed more or
less of our own free will. We do not have to smoke, drink, eat
excessively, engage in promiscuous sex, overdose on sun, and so
on. For most practical purposes we achieve step 1 in the cancer-
creating process by our own efforts. Remember also that while
many of us do smoke, drink, sunbathe and indulge excessively
in casual sex (and can therefore be said to be exposing ourselves
to step 1), not all of us develop cancer. Consequently, to look for
a personality type to link up with step 1, it must be someone
whose harmful behaviour is habitual.

Step 2 requires that the body's systems fail to react
adequately to damage, or if they do react, the effects are easily
overridden. In short any signs of discomfort caused by the
presence of the carcinogen are either *not* detected or they are
ignored. Translated into practical, everyday terms in relation to,
say, smoking, this means that for *step 2* to occur, you must systematically ignore your body's reactions to the presence of smoke. The
unpleasant taste and the irritability most people experience
when they first start smoking are gradually adjusted to so that
what orginally caused their systems to reject the foreign body
are now ignored in preference to a temporary feeling of pleasure.
Don't forget, nothing changes after that first experience of
smoking; your body's lower systems still react and register the
presence of a foreign agent and irritability; your higher systems
(in particular the central nervous system) become conditioned to
minimizing the lower alarm signals. Not only do they ignore
these signals, but the higher systems learn to want and expect

the presence of the agent. And in time an emotional chain becomes linked to smoking. Instead of the nervous system being alerted to the presence of irritation, certain parts of the system learn to relax in association with smoking. Endocrine patterns modify in line with this; you feel less stressed by the act of smoking and consequently your hormones transmit similar messages, according to your nervous systems' judgement of the situations. You can see that the degree to which this becomes ingrained in your pattern of living will determine your susceptibility to step 2.

Step 3 follows on from step 2. In order for the immune system to cope with the recurrent presence of a foreing body like smoke in the lungs, it requires the rest of the body support systems to support it. To provide a simple hypothetical example, take the immune reaction in the lung; obviously if an immune response is to work, in reaction to carcinogen-caused tissue changes, it will not want to be handicapped by the presence, say, of inadequate supplies of protein due to the inefficient action of the nervous and endocrine systems arising from step 2. Normal team work would have ensured that (a) the CNS would immediately abort the action of letting smoke into the lungs and (b) the endocrine system would have registered the need to act and supply the correct amount and balance of whatever the immune system needed. The collapse of this team work in any particular area leads eventually to the weakening of the immune system in that area.

Finally, this pattern of somatopsychic functioning must usually continue for a considerable length of time for it to be critical. The development of cancerous growths is generally extremely slow and we can infer that they occur as a result of long-standing poor team work in the body's reaction to the presence of low-level irritants. Another important point: if the irritant is major, most people will stop doing it smartly; it is the minor, apparently unimportant, day-to-day irritant, that is most likely to cause the vulnerabilities discussed above.

The key three-part sequence is laid down, or developed, in an adult's early twenties, developed that is, as a set of body behaviours and psychological attitudes to the body that remain fixed in place for the fifteen or twenty years it takes for a cancer to form. What matter are the habits that become an integral part of an individual's daily life and not temporary or casual habits suddenly adopted or discarded. In short we must look for a psychosomatic pattern that is well-supported by the individual's personality; that is, in fact, an integral part of his or her personality.

HOW TO THINK ABOUT THIS 3-STEP PROCESS

If you tend to think about your body as something separate from your mental or emotional activity you might be a little puzzled by my approach here. So far it all seems very straightforward and understandable; We are looking for the cause of cancer in terms of a set of quite ordinary actions which together, we think, do the damage. Moreover, those actions so far are explained as if they were simple, everyday events. It may seem as if cancer develops out of bad habits — habits you always meant to give up, but didn't — and eventually they harm you. In a sense this is true though somewhat simplistic. But we *can* look for how cancer starts in the day-to-day world in which we live. The origins of cancer lie in how we treat our bodies.

Most of us take our bodies pretty much for granted. As long as they seldom break down, we tend not to give them much thought. Indeed we are often indignant if internal goings-on intrude on our consciousness from time to time. When the body does pack up we become afraid, don't understand what's gone wrong, and view the malfunctioning body as some kind of inexplicable 'drag' on us.

Although what I have been saying about habits, overriding signals and lowering immunity might seem like alien concepts, understanding is closer at hand than you might think. Let's look at how you, the individual, have direct experience of your immune system. Take, for instance, starting a cold. Remember that period just before a cold begins? Haven't you ever felt that whether or not you do get a cold is somehow in your hands? Remember how sometimes you thought you were going to get one but didn't? Nine times out of ten, it was because something distracting cropped up, something demanded your attention and you forgot about the cold. Your alert psychological state boosted your immune system, allowing it to cope with the occurrence without going on full alert (which is when you actually get a cold). Team work; your CNS and your endocrine system acted to back the immune system before it was too late.

The 'something' that diverted your attention, be it a rush job at work which you just *had* to do, or a game of tennis you *had* to play, are the psychological equivalents of body events that alert your CNS and operate your endocrine system. You experience these events as psychological 'demands' which you obey, but your body experiences them as increased autonomic activity, as preparing the body for action (CNS activity) by pumping out adrenalin or growth hormone, making protein and energy available (endocrine activity). Your subjective experience is *equivalent* to the body experience. By pure chance – *having* to do a job, or play a game, or go on a date – at that time, your immune system needed the extra activity too; you coped with the cold purely as a by-product of having to do something else.

We can take this example a little further to see another important link. Research has established that you don't have to get colds; if you are psychologically attentive to your body, that is, if you take proper care especially when tired or upset, you will take steps to protect yourself; you'll sleep, eat properly, relax, break the strain, 'baby' yourself or whatever, and so help your immune system cope. There is nothing *physical* about this; it is a *psychological* step you take with physical consequences. If you fail to act, the immune system deteriorates slowly until it is gradually overwhelmed by a virus, say, that it could ordinarily keep under control and then ultimately sounds the alarm by *actually* registering all the unpleasant symptoms that we associate with a cold. At last, the immune system's messages get through to the brain and you register the need to do something. The point is that the immune system has been warning you all along but you, with your insensitivity to your body, overrode it. Eventually your immune system forces your mind (or central nervous system) to take the kind of protective steps it needs to combat the cold. You slow down, wrap up, take boosters and settle down to be miserable for a week. And for that week, at least, your mind is much more directly in touch with your immune system: it is in that state that you get some idea of the stress under which your body and the immune system has to operate. People who are chronically subject to colds are often found to be habitually unable to recognize their body signals.

Let me give you a few more examples of where I'm sure you have some subjective contact with your body systems. Take your endocrine system. If you're a man, imagine looking at or talking to an incredibly attractive woman; if you're a woman, imagine an incredibly attractive man. Think of all those feelings that flood the body: the dry throat, the tingling feeling, the rush of blood to your head, the feeling that the world has, for a moment, lurched to a stop. Your hormones are at work.

Another instance: imagine you're making love and you want to have an orgasm, but something goes wrong; you're interrupted, you lose the impulse or whatever. Remember that awful aching feeling of being stopped — that incredible let-down effect it has on your body? It's as if your endocrine system was suddenly thrown into reverse as indeed is the case. That subjective feeling is the mental equivalent to the body's reaction.

Another example: imagine someone has really upset you; you're incredibly angry, hurt and humiliated, but as you experience all this, you know there's absolutely nothing you can do about it, either because you don't have the power or they're not there. That feeling of intense body arousal with nowhere to go, like a bull stopped by a brick wall, is equivalent to the pressure on your body's endocrine and central nervous systems. Everything in you is ready to attack, or react, but is somehow prevented from doing so.

A last example: you want to relax. Let's say you want to get off to sleep, or you want to relax in a bath, or go to the toilet, but you can't – there's too much noise, you're scared of being disturbed, or heard. This is an instance of where the parasympathetic part of your central nervous system won't work properly. Your feeling tense is a subjective experience which exactly approximates that of your central nervous system.

Whenever you become excited, happy, tense or upset, all these psychological states correspond to equivalent states in the body. The *act* of being excited, or whatever, demands that the

body systems be in co-ordinated operation alongside your
subjective feeling; you can't *be* happy or sad or tense without
your body's systems. And the same goes for other states of mind
— being muddled, guilty, confused, irritable, puzzled, lethargic
and so on; they represent, as it were, thoughts of unease, when
you feel as if you're in two minds at once. And they have their
body system equivalents too; your CNS is in a state which is
half-active, half-passive; your endocrine system is unbalanced
and your immune system erratic.

It is very important that you appreciate just how integrated your mind and body are. From the moment you're born,
as you grow through childhood, you learn patterns of association, links between the body and mind and vice versa; everything you do has a subjective psychological part and a
body-state equivalent. How you walk, how you talk, how you
breathe, eat, sleep, interrelate, how you attend to your personal
hygiene, how you cope with problems, how you get upset, angry
and so on, all involve your mind *and* your body. If you talk
quietly or are shy, for example, the function of your vocal
chords, the position of your head, your body posture (a shy
posture is *physically* different to a challenging posture) become
linked in a behavioural chain that might start with the thought,
'I feel unsure of myself so I'll speak quietly in case I'm wrong',
but ends in a complex set of mental and physical interactions
that help to maintain the pattern. Our individuality and uniqueness as human beings is given (or arrived at) through the
accumulation of just these patterns.

This, of course, does not mean to suggest that everything is
'psychological'.

What I'm talking about is behaviour. We have to learn to
integrate our bodies and minds and we do this by activity,
behaviour. And as we act or behave (and remember, even
thinking or sleeping is an *action*) we create or perform sets of
interrelated body-mind links. There are, of course, times when
the body creates motives or needs that require attention, like
hunger, thirst, sleep and so on, which intrude on your mental
states. There are also times when purely mental events create a
need to act or react. When you suddenly remember you have to
do something you've forgotten, or if you decide after a lot of

thought to do something, you rouse your body and act. But these are incidental to the fact that as a growing individual, you carry out the actions as an integrated body-mind entity.

What really matters to us here is how this body-mind system works, how individual systems differ and above all, how specific kinds of body-mind integrations are linked to diseases like cancer. Many of the theories that have arisen this century about cancer have not, in fact, looked at the individual and his/her body in this way. They have focused, with rare exceptions, either on the body or on the mind as separate entities. Thus some theories have seen cancer as arising purely as a result of some failure in the *body*. Other theories have seen it as a failure in the *mind*: aggression unexpressed, perhaps, or a vulnerable, repressed personality without any real understanding of quite why this should result in cancer when the same 'psychological' cause is also said to account for drug addiction or schizophrenia. These are reductionistic, over-simplified theories; we will focus instead on the body-mind system of behaviour that characterizes individuals who develop cancer.

What we want to see is the way in which a person's general behaviour can be related to the criteria we have set up for the formation of cancer. Let's return once again to the three-step process. However, this time, we want to spell out what each of the steps means in terms of body-mind behaviours.

Expanding step 1: The carcinogen factor   Most of the high risk carcinogens are ingested, or we are exposed to them, through our own actions. How could this be done in such a fashion as to predispose someone to cancer? One case in point is when this occurs routinely: chronic smokers, for example, chronic sunbathers, people who consistently eat large quantities of food thought to contain carcinogens, people who are prone to constipation and retain food for too long in their intestines. The links are there, as we saw earlier but on their own they can't account for cancer in individual cases. We know that lung cancer incidence has risen in proportion to the number of people smoking. We know that constipated Westerners are more likely to get colorectal cancer than far less-constipated Africans. We know that skin cancer rates are highest in sunny places.

Does this mean that smoke, diet and sun cause cancer? Or does it mean that how particular individuals use smoking, how they actually suntan or how and what they eat causes cancer?

Where you live and the cultural and social circumstances you live in set up certain predisposing patterns. Thus, if you live in a culture that supports a certain kind of behaviour – smoking, eating in particular ways, suntanning – and that behaviour can be engaged in easily or freely, then these influences can be said to key the direction cancer is likely to take. Arctic Eskimoes aren't liable to get cancer from over-suntanning; similarly, if you live in a non-smoking community, cigarettes will not key you to lung cancer.

At best your culture is going to set a direction for any possible cancer depending on the kind of tolerance it has for any given carcinogens. The carcinogen is unlikely on its own to give you cancer; as significant is the individual's style of indulgence. Take tobacco smoking: do we all smoke in the same way? Clearly not; practically everyone who smokes does so in his or her own manner. There are light smokers and heavy smokers, but some 'light' smokers inhale deeply, some don't. Some 'heavy' smokers don't inhale much. In fact, a case has recently been made out that lighter smokers might have an inhalation pattern that puts them more at risk than heavier smokers.

Similarly, some occasional smokers only smoke after meals. Other occasional smokers only smoke between meals. Each pattern can have a different effect; ingesting tobacco on an empty stomach is different in a number of ways from smoking on a full stomach.

Take this a step further. Most smokers start to smoke for reasons that have little to do with the desire to taste smoke. Teenagers and schoolchildren might do so out of a sense of breaking the rules, of being part of a gang. Many people start to smoke in social situations, as a prop to help them be, or seem to be, like other people. Some people smoke when they're socially anxious because it gives them something to do with their hands. They 'feel' more at ease; standing at a cocktail party awkwardly without a cigarette somehow highlights their anxiety (they think). Other people smoke, not to break anxiety, but to break their concentration, just as someone else might have a cup of coffee or tea.

We are all individuals. If we are all exposed to the same cultural carcinogen pattern (as by and large we are) then how we actually use this exposure will vary from person to person. We smoke, eat, sleep, drink, make love, all in highly specific ways. Take eating, for example. It does more than simply satisfy a basic hunger; it is intimately bound up with our senses of self, with our security, with our anxiety, our feeling of being alive and so on. Most of us do much *more* than eat in order to stop feeling hungry; we eat too much, or too little, we eat little delicacies, we eat mush, or whatever makes us feel *nice* as well as full. We eat sometimes to alleviate anxiety, we eat sometimes to take our minds off things. We use meal times in important social ways, as means of sharing time and communications.

Given all this individual variation, you can see that saying something like 'cigarette smoking causes cancer' is too simple. We need to specify the *way* in which, for example, an individual smokes, before we can advance our understanding of how any carcinogen can be linked to the cancer-prone person. Of all the individuals who smoke or eat the wrong sort of food, or otherwise expose themselves to carcinogens, what behaviour pattern will ensure the kind of exposure to a carcinogen which creates the first of our cancer-inducing steps?

Perhaps the best way to characterize the habits I have in mind is to describe them simply as over-indulgences. There is nothing weird about cancer-inducing habits. Mostly they are normal, culturally-tolerated ways of behaving, which we all indulge in from time to time. The difference between the habits of the individual who becomes a cancer risk and someone who does not lies in the attitude each takes towards the irritant. Look, again, at smoking. There are many ways that smoking can be performed in relative safety. If, for example, you smoke to relieve your nervousness at a social function, you can be said to be using smoking as a catalyst to help you cope. Like all catalysts, it serves or should serve an end beyond itself. Once you feel relaxed, you should not need to smoke. If you smoke, and either don't relax but nevertheless go on smoking out of habit, or if you *do* relax but smoke on anyway, you're pushing the original function beyond its limits. You're exposing yourself to step 1.

Society tolerates smoking and in doing so it keys the individual to certain cancers. However society has no means of teaching moderation or appropriate use and so while the individual is free to use it in the right context, the right time and place and to monitor his or her body reaction, the opposite applies equally.

Take a second example. Most people today, especially in adolescence and early adulthood, engage in sexual relations as a means of making intimate contact with someone. It is often used, in these early exploratory stages, as a clumsy, sometimes crude means of discovering yourself, how to channel your feelings and how to care in turn for another. It is also, often, distressing. You may feel guilty, 'dirty' and repulsive, as well as excited. Sex at this time is a catalyst; it helps a person grow up, it is a means to an end. You should go beyond it to discover real, emotional and psychological intimacy with another person and to deepen and broaden your own and the other's sexual enjoyment. It should become, in short, an integral part of living.

When, however, the act retains its adolescent connotations leaving you feeling ugly and unfulfilled, and if you continue to abuse sex by sleeping with a number of different partners without proper intimacy developing, then the habit is not serving its proper function. Research has established that people who frequently change sex partners expose themselves to infections which can be carcinogenic. Moreover, enjoying healthy integrated sex brings with it sets of relaxed habits which ensure low exposure to carcinogens; if you feel good about sex, you will respond more fully in the act, be less open to physical hurt, or irritation through dryness, and your personal cleanliness will be better — all important in cutting down exposure to carcinogens.

When you find that you're using a habit for its own ends alone and doing it routinely, then you are running risks. And it can be as simple as eating too much chocolate; it's lovely to eat chocolate and it gives you energy too, but some people daily gorge on huge quantities of it because they like the satisfaction it gives. When it is blown out of all proportion, when it replaces other more fulfilling actions to become an end itself, then you may be approaching step one.

Many personal habits can assume these proportions. It is very likely that a great many people expose themselves poten-tially to cancer at this level by using perfectly mundane habits – eating, drinking, smoking, masturbating, making love, scratch-ing, sunbathing – in the wrong ways. That is, they use the habit as an end in itself or they persist in a behaviour without it being used as a building block to better psychological things. As we said earlier, this probably results in the pre-cancerous conditions which are destroyed by the body's system before they become malignant. More is needed before the transformation into cancer actually takes place.

Expanding step 2: The central nervous and endocrine factors

Many of us, as part of our daily lives, engage in *step 2* habits. That is, we don't react appropriately to discomfort or body stress, especially if the stressed state is at a low level. Think of playing a game of football or tennis, when you injure a muscle painfully. You know that for your body's sake you should stop and nurse the muscle at least for a while. But equally, you're in a game, the muscle is not too sore, you can override the pain. So you do; you play on until the game is finished. We all do it; in fact, we admire people who do it, who keep going even though injured, hurt or in discomfort. As growing boys and girls, we're taught how admirable ignoring pain is: our heroes push themselves beyond limits which would make most of us scream. We teach this notion at all social levels and in extremely thorough ways.

There's the 'Indiana Jones' type of override, the 'famous explorer' type, the 'super-athlete' type, there's even the 'rock guitarist' type — playing when fingers are bleeding and dehydration threatens from losing so much sweat. And then there's the 'super-workaholic' type who pushes his or her body through hell to get things done; the writer who turns out huge quantities of material against all odds; the good doctor who gets three hours' sleep a night but believes he is doing such important work it doesn't matter.

There's nothing wrong with overriding. Indeed *constructive* overriding is an important part of making your body and your mind healthy. Every time you take a little exercise, every time you have to think a bit harder about something, you're using override to stretch your body systems, to make them perform just a little bit more. Overriding is a catalyst too. You can use override to great effect; you can stretch your body physically and psychologically in ways which if used to achieve some worthwhile end, can be very useful to you. Provided override is used with care, never as an end in itself, and you take the right precautions to compensate afterwards, nothing should go wrong. The point is that like everything else, override has to be used or learned in an appropriate context. Out of context, problems occur. Let's look at normal versus abnormal patterns of over-riding and you'll see what I mean.

Normal overriding   At birth, we are very simple entities. Much of what happens to babies, in the behavioural sense, is physically or biologically determined with practically no role for conscious, higher-level thinking, or directing. There is no question initially of override. A baby sleeps, wees, burps, cries, smiles and demands food in regular patterns dictated by his or her basic physiological requirements. The baby's body systems have to act on only the most basic needs. This is, of course, very necessary for the baby; its endocrine, central nervous and immune systems are immature and need this protective simplicity in order to develop and mature. As the child grows, it begins to extend its systems. Growth of consciousness, growth of awareness alert the child to the world outside its body. It has limits — feeding time, the edge of the cot, time with its parents — and the child naturally begins to explore these as well as its own bodily and movement limits. The act of exploration is a vital part of growth; the child learns to link conscious feelings to physical and movement sensations, to a whole range of experiences. And as it does this, it grows as a body-mind entity.

Gradually however, the growing child learns to recognize two very different sets of demands. The first, the most familiar, are the needs to eat, drink, sleep, rest, explore, urinate, defecate, cry, smile and so on. Imposed on these are the second demands from parents and the environment; to eat at a set time, in a set

way, with set food, to sleep at a set time, to go to the toilet, to
cry, smile, explore. ... all at set times and in set ways. Inevitably, override occurs; a child has to learn to wait, to be less
'impulsive', sometimes not to act out at all. He or she has to learn
to regiment many body signals and needs. But ideally, this
always occurs in a useful context. The child learns, for instance,
to control an urge to urinate and does so in the knowledge that
the urge *will* be satisfied soon; that there is a time and place.
Learning this means-end behaviour lays the foundation for
much of what we call normal overriding; you learn first to
register the body signals, but not to follow through the baby-
immediate action chain and then, second, you learn to express
your need in a socially acceptable manner, i.e. the child will say
to mum or dad, 'Look, can we find a toilet'. Thirdly, you will
eventually learn to deal with your needs appropriately yourself,
i.e. you'll find somewhere to relieve yourself.

This learning of appropriate override behaviour patterns is
an incredibly important and thorough-going process. It is a vital
part of developing a healthy body and mind and it normally
applies to every level of functioning. You learn these patterns
first and most basically at home from your parents and your
family; as you grow and venture more into the outside world,
you learn sets of more sophisticated override habits, at school,
with your friends, in business, or your job, with your life
partners. At school you learn for example, patterns of working;
you learn that to pass exams you have to work hard and push
yourself. You learn to go without sleep and rest for appropriate
ends, you learn to override fatigue or eye strain. If you play
sport, you learn to override pain, as discussed earlier.

Faulty overriding   Now let's see where this can go wrong. We
can identify three basic growing levels; the transition from baby
needs to family-orientated needs, i.e. learning to override and
contextualize your basic physiological requirements; the transition from family-override habits to those imposed by the outside
world; and lastly the transition from this state to the full, adult
level of habit where *you* yourself set and limit your override
behaviours. Problems can arise at each level.

At the first level, at home, you can learn to override habits

that interfere too much with the proper or appropriate fulfil-
ment of your body (or baby) needs. There are certain pre-
requisites for fulfilling basic needs comfortably. For example, if
you eat under pressure or under anxiety, you don't swallow or
chew properly, you don't digest properly, you don't eat the right
food, or approach eating in the right context. Anorexia and
indigestion are just some of the obvious and familiar results, but
there are others. Eating with anxiety (a menacing or hostile
father or mother ramming food into your mouth) disrupts the
normal pattern of smooth CNS-endocrine functioning; anxiety
and stress release stress hormones into the blood which interfere
with the body's job of changing the food into protein. Anxiety
interferes with the CNS's autonomic relaxation processes; food
is thus poorly absorbed and remains too long in the stomach,
causing discomfort, some of which you can feel. But when it
occurs as a routine, automatic part of your life, you condition
your body to ignore the feelings. Eventually you believe that this
pattern is normal. We're talking about low-level discomfort that
easily gets lost in the acts of coping with meal times, or the
family.

We can examine each area of body functioning and find
similar vital chains. Going to the toilet should be an anxiety-free
activity with your body feeling quite relaxed, with plenty of time to
perform. Your body needs this relaxation to urinate or defecate
properly. Having someone banging on the door, watching you,
pressurizing you, cutting your time down, interferes with this.
You may become constipated, or incontinent, or you may
develop bad cleaning habits — all in the interests of relieving
anxiety. These seemingly minor reactions become problematic
over time. We will look at each body system in more detail in
Chapter 4.

Let me emphasize that these are routine, daily levels of
activity to which you become adjusted for which you have
developed an inappropriate override habit. In short, you learn to
ignore or put up with your own discomfort in favour of pleasing
or conforming to someone else's demand. It is low level, true, but
we are only interested, remember, in low-level routines just like
these. One other point. It is rare for a single individual to have
faulty override habits in every area of functioning; usually only

one or two areas are affected, but it does mean that the poor habit creates a weakness in body-mind functioning in that area – a vulnerability that can contribute to putting you at risk in the second step of getting cancer.

When one goes to school, one faces fresh override demands. Depending on early training in the home, the demands at this higher level can make matters worse (or better). Adulthood brings with it many new demands and returns you in a way to some older ones; in particular, intimacy can re-awaken old problems or levels of functioning that adolescence and school obscured.

An adult faces a lot of pressures. Becoming an individual is no easy task. Clearly adult overrides will be coped with better if basic, baby-body needs were well-managed, i.e. leaving few vulnerabilities from earlier stages and if the body and mind's override abilities are properly learned. Unfortunately, being an adult, holding down a job, and having a spouse and family, creates a lot of new demands, leaving little time to change any earlier patterns. Once you've got them, by and large, you keep them. And often they are compounded. Alcohol and cigarettes used for social relaxation are often new and fun ways for young adults to solve long-standing anxiety and self-confidence problems.

How faulty override habits can lead to cancer-proneness in step 2   For your body and its systems to function properly it needs to be used – to be exercised, challenged, provoked and so on to fulfil the job for which it is designed. Ideally this means that all levels should be routinely operating in a full, contextual cycle. If you run, you must also rest; if you really push yourself to solve a problem, you must rest your mind once you've solved it. These cycles, called basic rest-activity cycles, are the patterns of behaviour that ensure healthy body-mind function and they are comprehensive. It is as important to push your mind in cycles as it is to exercise; it is as important to push your emotions through the correct cycles as it is to sleep properly, and so on. Remember, even though you mature and grow up, your baby needs still remain with you. We can understand these baby needs regarding eating and sleeping, but they also apply to emotions like happiness, sadness, and anger. Put it this way: a baby expresses itself and operates its body very efficiently. It cries in the right places (for it), laughs, grabs and squeezes, its nervous system and endocrine system being in almost perfect co-ordination. It is very important to cry if you are upset and to shout or be cross when you're angry – just as important as sleeping when you're tired, or emptying your bowels when they're full. Doing this ensures that the body systems work in proper co-ordination. Arousal taking place when you're angry. Crying relaxes you and lets your body unwind after it has been stressed. These are natural rest-activity cycles in which the healthy override gives way to the proper, contextual rest phase. Context, incidentally, is a key word – it means the right time and place for you. We'll go into it more later. Cycles like this ensure that your CNS and endocrine systems are working effectively both as a team and individually. The CNS needs arousal-rest sequences to work properly, otherwise nervous and muscle tensions develop and it throws out lower level operations; stomach, breathing and digestive functions work under-par. The endocrine system requires the right sequence to allow its hormones and steroids to do their work; it's no good pumping the body full of adrenalin and then not letting the rest phase or the action phase take place properly — you leave the body alert and aroused for too long and lethargy, loss of energy and tiredness follow.

A cancer risk person, therefore, would be someone whose override habits result in one or all of the following patterns:

The override is applied in the wrong areas   Instead of the override being used where healthy activity is engaged in, the person overrides discomfort and pain in areas that should not be so tolerated, in particular, smoking, eating, digestion, evacuation, love-making habits, where the risks of contact with carcinogens or irritation are high. This is made worse if the override is well-established and has become an integral part of daily life.

The person uses override in certain areas so much that not only are the behaviours liable to be contorted, but actually cease to exist   Some people, as they grow up, are pressured not to show emotion, not to cry, not to be angry, not to be self-orientated, not to be needy, dependent and so on. If these demands are rigorously enforced (or the behaviours too strongly punished) the individual stops the behaviour as the safest way of surviving. Stopping the expression of vital CNS-endocrine actions, such as crying when upset, can cause many disturbances.

Normal override habits are avoided   Some people avoid pushing themselves or their bodies through normal ranges of activity: they do not play sport, exercise, use their minds, have relationships, express emotions or make love. A few people avoid all such habits, others engage very minimally. Both result in under-development of body-mind systems and can create vulnerability if the individual is suddenly faced with a crisis.

None of these circumstances on their own cause cancer. Even taken together, i.e. if you engage in all three, there is no guarantee you'll develop cancer. However, the more your behaviour conforms with the above three phases, the greater the risk of increasing your proneness to cancer, especially if you also qualify under *step 1*. You might, for example, use override in the wrong way at certain times, but also have long periods when you use normal override too. This accounts for the person who has occasional problems with eating, indigestion, constipation, and so on. The risk is there but it stays low because the dangerous pattern does not become a routine one. It is broken up by healthy periods which give the body a chance to function normally.

Similarly, some people live on even though they might avoid or be afraid of any kind of body-mind challenge; inevitably, in my experience, these are protected people who, either through fortuitous circumstance or having very supportive relationships, have their particular needs met. Again, these people can suddenly find themselves at enormous risk if their protective systems are removed or lost.

Unfortunately, the three override patterns do tend to go together; override is applied in the wrong area, specific central body-mind behaviours are repressed and normal overrides avoided. When this happens too much, so that a routine pattern evolves over many years, you enter *step 2* and become cancer-prone. You create a CNS-endocrine vulnerability that is often specific to one area of the body. When combined with *step 1*, your body cannot register information and organize itself properly to cope with the damage. You become vulnerable to cancer through this omission. You do not have cancer yet, but you're well on the way; only one more step needs to take place.

Expanding step 3: The immune factor   Are there sets of habits, or behaviours, that lead to lowered levels of immunity? I distinguish between the routine ups and downs, daily fluctuations that our bodies normally exhibit and the imposition through habit of a generalized low level of immune action, one that has particular relevance for tumours. Are there specific behaviours that decrease our ability to cope with tumours? It's not that the immune system *causes* cancer, but after *steps 1 and 2* have become routine, after cancer cells have been created and are set to proliferate, *then*, in sequence, the immune system fails to stop them.

The answer to the question above is 'yes'. Very recently, research has identified sets of behaviours that have been linked to the immune system's tumour-surveillance function. One set of studies has been looking closely at the links between natural killer cell activity (NKCA) — a newly-discovered immune cell in the body that identifies and kills cancer cells — and various measures of psychological functioning and stress. It has been found that people who experience anxiety and stress on a routine, day-to-day level tend to have persistently lower NKCA measures than people who don't experience high levels of anxiety. The argument here is that poor coping with stress (we all experience stress, but some people don't let it get them down) lowers the level of the immune system and this over time can create a chronic vulnerability to growths. This *long-term pattern*, rather than stress on its own, bears a relationship to low levels of NKCA.

Interestingly enough, among the test findings, a factor called *interpersonal sensitivity* has one of the highest correlations with decreased NKCA; this, together with reports of significant correlations between the experience of anxiety, depression and a tendency to be obsessive-compulsive creates the picture of an individual whose habits revolve around feeling insecure, unsure of him- or herself, and a tendency to act out of fear rather than excitement or a desire to explore. In a study done in America, it was found that people with this kind of habitual attitude to life were twice as likely to die from cancer as those without it. Studies of widowers and widows following the death of their spouses have consistently shown that the resultant general pattern of depressed functioning seriously lowers the level of functioning of the immune system. Inability to cope with shock and loneliness are also often mentioned in this context. Significantly, too, in other studies, notably by a Columbus, Ohio team, chronic loneliness combined with high stress have been shown to be related to NKCA.

Still to be decided by research is the vital question: how do these patterns work to lower immunity? One argument is that the feelings of isolation, loneliness and depression tend to encourage other behaviours, like smoking, drinking, poor eating habits, and so on as a means of filling the emotional gaps inside. And it is these that actually lower the body's resistance. However, it seems to me that there is a more direct link between the two levels.

Much of the research on brain or CNS-immune links has been able to show that immune responses not only vary with psychological state, but that the operation of the immune system may depend in part on the keying action of the CNS. From birth the behaviour between parents and child acts to set up specific patterns in which these links are established. The child who can run to mum or dad for cuddles and reassurance if not feeling well is a child who will learn an easy pattern of recognizing and reporting changes in his or her body. Simple conditioning will create the same internal links as it learns from its parents; his or her CNS will be sensitive to immune needs and he/she will comfort or attend to itself. Self-comforting, self-cuddling are the in-between stages of learning proper CNS-immune links. In fact, several studies have shown how effectively the immune system can be conditioned to psychological events.

Lastly, other research has shown that there are definite organic links between the CNS and the immune system. We know that the communication links between mind and all levels of body occur at every level of action; it is now a matter of working out precisely how these links are tied into the CNS and how they are changed or controlled by mind-body behaviour. Let me present what we know in a simplified form as I'm sure it will help you recognize the pattern.

Most people express worry or distress by moaning or complaining and getting upset. Healthy behaviour involves a high level of mind-body integration, and unhealthy behaviour a very low level of mind-body interaction. Healthy people, for example, become upset in a way that actually helps them. Usually they have someone they can turn to for comfort or reassurance. Less-healthy people also express their upset, but they do it in unproductive ways; they might become *too* upset, collapse, get hysterical, become over-dependent and demanding, or equally harmful, pretend nothing is wrong. Far less healthy people don't express their upset directly to anyone – they do it indirectly: drive too fast, drink too much, break things, be self-destructive, and so on, until someone takes notice, or something goes wrong.

As we go down the behaviour scale, each worsening step means less proper psychological contact is made with a person outside yourself. Distress is directly translated into low-level body function without being communicated to another person. Someone who fits this category, for example, might feel sick, upset, get dizzy or have headaches. These are often the only means he or she knows of showing upset. A healthy person recognizes body distress signs immediately, knows what they mean and finds a way of first expressing them and then doing something about the problem. The body systems aren't used except as a means of relief, such as crying in someone's arms. Less-healthy people don't recognize that their bodies are signalling stress (they override the signs) and they won't act until the tension registers as head pain, nausea or whatever. Evidence shows that unsatisfactory though this pattern may be, it is not linked to lowered immunity in the sense of lowered NKCA.

Individuals who neither use other people, nor psycho-somatic symptoms as a means of reacting to stress are, however, using patterns linked to lowered immunity. Instead, distressed, they simply slump physiologically. They carry on at whatever their role demands; they don't show their upset to anyone, they don't stop, don't get sick and certainly don't get hypochon-driacal. They simply become resigned, feel helpless — 'what's the use' — put their heads down and lower their immunity. They are so conditioned *not* to act on their body's signals of distress that they miss vital early signs, and don't help them-selves even when the problem is low-key. They do this as a rou-tine, everyday matter-of-course. Normally, if you are tense, for example, and develop a headache, the headache forces you to slow your body down, take rest and this helps the body cope. If you're tense but so conditioned to ignore it, the tension becomes a fixed part of your body's internal environment. Getting a headache at least ensures the tension will eventually be dissi-pated.

The cancer-prone pattern we're examining ensures a chronic override of body sounds plus the presence of relatively chronic tension in one form or another. Little or no relief ever seems to occur and it is this pattern that is associated with lowered immunity and step 3 cancer risk.

PUTTING THE CANCER HABITS TOGETHER

Life would be much simpler if there were one such straight-forward thing as a cancer-prone personality. There are, it's true, some personality traits that are linked to cancer people which we'll come to shortly, but knowing them doesn't help much. For one thing, there isn't an actual *personality* type. There isn't any *one* thing that marks you down for cancer. There isn't any one psychological pattern anymore than there is any *one* cell or germ that gives you cancer. It is more complicated than that. Getting cancer is a matter of how you *behave* and that involves how you, as a body-mind entity, act as a whole.

The three-step way of thinking about getting cancer says that you need all three events before a cell becomes a malignant tumour. Having two or one won't do — you might carry nearly-cancerous cells around with you, but you'd be safe.

We need a model that accounts for the enormous variability of cancer. Why does it suddenly strike some people and grow very fast? Why do others get it and then it goes away? Why are many cancers very slow in their growth rates? How can we get cancer on a daily basis and eliminate it equally on a daily basis? Or not? Why do some people get cancer at some times but not others? If we look for answers to these questions at the purely psychological level or at the purely organic level, we get only partial answers. There is no set cancer personality; cancer victims vary enormously in their personalities. We can't identify actual, specific psychological traits that guarantee cancer. Similarly, there is no cancer germ, no actual carcinogen, no chemical that *always* causes cancer.

We can answer the questions, though, if we focus on the *behaviour* of the body-mind system as a whole. And we can do that because the behavioural chain we have described and which causes cancer, is a flexible, complex model. It is a model that not only focuses on the biopsychological entity that the human is, but allows for interactions between the elements of the chain.

Consider this: let's say you as a general rule definitely exhibit habits that expose you to *step 3* risk. Let's say you're a depressive, inert sort of person who definitely has lowered resistance. Your NKCA count is low. Will you get cancer? No. Not unless you also are at risk from *steps 1 and 2* habits. That is, you'd have to also expose yourself to carcinogens regularly *and* override your body signals in the wrong way. If your immunity was low, but you ate the right food, slept, drank, and performed your body functions well, had no pain or discomfort, didn't smoke or drink much, especially not in distress, you'd probably survive.

To take a second example, you are at risk from *step 1*. You smoke heavily, drink a lot, eat junk food, work in an asbestos factory and sniff furniture glue as a hobby; will you get cancer? No. Not unless you also are at risk from *steps 2 and 3* — that is, if you override wrongly, and have chronically lowered immunity. Some people, heavy smokers exposed to carcinogens, for example, may lead quite healthy lives otherwise; they exercise, play sport, laugh, cry, enjoy themselves, go to bed early, stop smoking the moment they get a cold, and so on, and it is these habits that protect them from developing a tumour. The carcinogen may damage cells, small malignant growths might occur, but they are taken care of by the team work of the rest of the body's systems.

It's all a question of timing and balance. It is possible, for example, for a person to be exposed to all three risks at the same time without cancer occurring; providing the occasions are of short duration and don't happen too often. Some people, therefore, can develop cancer but then break the pattern and recover. By the same token, some people lead apparently healthy lives, but then are suddenly exposed to all the risks at the same time — usually when they are at a very vulnerable age — and cancer starts. I'm thinking here of cancer in young children, cancer in those suddenly losing a job, their spouses, or who otherwise undergo massive unwelcome changes.

Other people might be exposed routinely to *steps 1 and 2*, but through living in a particular way or in a particular relationship, avoid *step 3*. Subtle changes in living patterns might expose them to *step 3* and cancer starts. If the balance of an individual's habits changes, even subtly, the chain is completed.

The model provides for variations in habits and in this way accounts for the variable forms cancer takes. It permits us to identify those behaviours that make up the risk chain and thus we can finally identify the overall pattern that puts any given individual at serious risk. You can be sure that if your behaviour falls into all three steps at the same time and this persists as a routine for many years, you'll suffer cancer. Let's now focus on these habits as a group and identify the psychological links that accompany them.

THE PSYCHOLOGY OF HIGH-RISK INDIVIDUALS

What we're going to do now is look at the *worst-case* pattern and identify the psychological framework associated with those behaviours.

You might be surprised how closely the research reports of

the kind of psychological patterns associated with cancer-prone people fit into the model I have presented. You'll recall that overall, four areas of psychological relevance were consistently found in cancer-prone people: a disturbance in family background, a disturbance in parent-child relationships, a disturbance in interpersonal relationships, and a disturbance in coping behaviour. Care must be taken, though, in incorporating these findings into our *worst-case* model. Let's therefore take a growing child who develops cancer as an adult and examine the psychological world in which he or she learns to live. Much of what follows is an amalgam of my own research on family life of cancer victims and the findings reported in Chapter 2.

The early years   As you grow up, where do you learn your habits? This simple-to-answer question is nevertheless of vital importance because while we all know that most of our habits are learned at home, in the family, few of us realize how deeply ingrained these domestic habits become in our day-to-day adult living. There are whole sets of behaviours we take for granted without realizing where we learned them — or, that there may be other ways of performing them. How we brush our teeth, chew food, go to the toilet, wash, when we change our clothes and so on, are all learned at home. In fact, much of our basic learning from *day one* in life occurs in the context of relationships, which is one reason why relationships figure so prominently in psychology of cancer research.

As you grow you need to develop all aspects of you. The baby, remember, is an almost perfect body-mind entity. A healthy adult is one who has been permitted to develop all aspects of body-mind functioning in a co-ordinated, systematic way. The growing baby or child needs to explore, to be 'childish', to be crude in its actions, thoughts and feelings. It must be able to make mistakes, to be gently guided (sometimes firmly), so that it can build on what it finds, learn to link actions and results, with body sensations, thoughts, and movements and so on. Its body has to be used, its muscles stretched, its needs fulfilled in healthy ways; it has to be given the freedom to make the vital links needed by the body-mind networks to arrive at properly integrated behaviour. This is especially so in two areas of functioning: emotions and internal body activity, or *body awareness*. Take, for instance, getting upset. A child has a fright, he or she experiences a whole rush of internal body states corresponding to the emotions. They create a massive need for which something must be done, some action taken. A normal child automatically shows fear, takes evasive action and runs for cover or comfort. A normal parent will build on these automatic reactions and will acknowledge the fear, accept and even encourage the tears, provide the physical contact needed for security and protection and take the time to look at the whole event, thus reassuring the child. This simple act ensures that a whole chain of vital body-mind interactions are learned; the child learns to cry, to run for help, to be comforted, learns to face the fear again, to repeat the process, and so on. All ensure the internal body pressure is released, allowing the body cycle to go through its arousal-expression-rest state. Above all though, the child learns that (a) it has the right to impose on its parents, and (b) it has the right to have its own world-view attended to. Both ensure that the child views its own world and its own body actions in *security*. It does not have to be afraid and alone. Now, imagine what happens if this process is stopped; if the child is ignored by the parent, told to shut up, told to behave, to avoid the upsetting situation, or worse, is punished for being a nuisance. Even worse it might receive apparently 'correct support' but sense the adult's irritation with it. Imagine this as a routine in specific areas day in and day out — what does the child do?

Most normal children will learn to avoid needing the parent's help, will find someone else for support, or will cope on their own. What seems to happen in cancer-prone people, though, is that the parent's reaction is so severe it actually causes more distress and anxiety than the original incident. After this has happened a few times, the child learns two basic habits; to avoid anything like the original incident *and* to avoid showing the behaviour which upset the parent.

The result is that the child still gets upset (it's difficult to avoid upsetting incidents), but systematically refuses to attend to its upset which means that it won't show distress, won't act on body sensation and won't turn to anyone else. The evidence is that in this latter area the cancer victim is most at risk; if a child *can* find someone else and can continue growing in these areas, learning can continue. The crippling aspect of the parent-child relationship for the cancer-prone person is that learning to turn to someone else does not occur either. In a sense we can say that the growing child slowly becomes conditioned not to seek comfort, not to use others and ultimately, not to develop the necessary language about inner distress and discomfort that an ordinary child does.

The problem for the growing cancer-prone child is that this emotional curtailment affects his or her ability to cope with stress in other areas of development. If you have never been permitted to express internal distress you never learn through experience to develop the behaviours, internal connections and inter-personal connections necessary for body survival. Consequently, when it comes to dealing with anything that triggers off these internal upsets, you will always react in the same way, never progressing. The older you grow, the more difficult it becomes to go through the necessary learning experiences, and the undeveloped part of you remains fixed. You remain almost entirely dependent on the more powerful in your world to help you through emotional or stressful episodes.

It is worth pausing here and thinking about what this actually means. Most of us take for granted how we perceive our internal body states. Most of us are so used to taking time to look after ourselves that we have no idea what it would be like to put up with daily pain, irritation and stress, only getting relief when someone outside did something about it. Most of us have *private time* to attend to our own needs. We expect *peace* and *quiet* in order to listen to what's going on in our bodies, to reflect, act and decide what to do. Imagine never learning this, never taking it for granted. Without this time we still experience the pain, discomfort and stress but we learn to live with it, as a nuisance that we hope will go away. Imagine having a stomach ache, but not having the time to *feel* the pain, to *stop* what you're doing and wait till the pain's over. Imagine not knowing that it's okay to double over, to cry out or collapse. Imagine not having the sense of personal *freedom* to try different tactics to ease the pain, such as lying down, vomiting or going to the toilet.

Much of our healthy normal *growing time* is spent on learning how to cope with stress and pain, anxiety and upset, by minimizing the discomfort through body actions and mental tricks.

I found that the early lives of cancer people were so focused on what their parents were doing or needed that there was never time (or the place) for their own needs, nor for learning how to protect themselves. As one of my patients put it:

> 'If I got a stomach ache or something, it just had to wait. I would usually be too busy, too engrossed in family matters. And also, I was the "good" child; I tried never to get sick, not like my brother. He was a real cry baby.'

The actual reason for this state of affairs varied from family to family; sometimes, as in Karin's case, a demanding brother took up most of her mother's and father's time; in others it was a sick parent, sometimes it was neither, but the child felt that his or her parents' lives were so tense or fragile that he or she didn't want to add to the problems.

The key psychological states that need to be developed in this early stage of growth to ensure high cancer risk can thus be summed up as follows:

- The child over-focuses on the world *outside* itself. It becomes too 'real', too attentive to the demands of the people or events in the family.
- The child neglects its own experiences both in terms of its own bodily needs, and its own emotional needs.
- The child learns to tolerate high levels of discomfort, stress and pain. It has no sense of personal body-mind time or rights.
- The child lacks adequate emotional development and this is shown in an inability to manage or express upset or stress properly, either mentally or physically.
- The child is too tied to the learned family pattern, and cannot (through being discouraged or not knowing how) get help in outside relationships, so little or no emotional learning takes place.

- The child learns the family's pattern of stress management. Usually this takes two forms: presenting a bland indifference when upset – 'Everything goes still and quiet inside — I just wait for it to pass' – and a tendency to seek relief in routine and rituals like smoking, eating, repeating clichés, sleeping, and so on.
- The child learns to perceive itself as a vulnerable person in a vulnerable family at constant risk from the outside world. Parents who cannot accept emotions in their children are themselves emotionally frozen and inevitably cope with stressful but normal life events as if they were major crises when they're not. This frightens the child and helps confirm the child's inattention to self-needs. Ideally the growing child needs to be insulated from the outside world and exposed to it slowly.

From school to adulthood　So long as the child reared in the above fashion stays within the family, the risks of disturbance remain low. For one thing the child does not expect to cope with normal ups and downs; it knows that it can turn to mother or father for practically everything. Most parents of my cancer patients were actually caring people and did 'look after' their children in the simple sense of providing for their basic material needs. However, once outside the protective family, cancer-prone people run into trouble. Unable to cope with stress and not knowing how to learn to cope, they feel terribly vulnerable. They are unable to use other people (friends, teachers and the like), unable (nor permitted) to express distress, and create the *impression* of coping by their calm and apparently relaxed exteriors. Homelife becomes all important as the growing person puts increasingly greater pressure on parents to provide reassurance and security.

As the growing individual's exposure to the real world increases, so does his exposure to stressful situations. Exams, challenges, demands and sports are aimed at him or her personally, no longer at the family; he or she is not expected to rely on mother or father and consequently finds the internal pressures mounting. Trying to get help from home inevitably results in the parents' distancing themselves in subtle but key ways; they now regard the growing child as a demanding source of distress to them and they hold back which, I think, results in the finding reported in many studies of distance and a lack of warmth from their families felt by cancer victims.

The adolescent thus finds him or herself alone and ill-equipped to cope with the world, and it is at this time, I feel, that conditioned helplessness as a survival pattern becomes firmly established in the cancer-prone individual. Without the protection and learning offered by the original parental relationship, the individual *is* in fact helpless. Faced with stress or with the need to cope or express emotions the individual retreats into the bland, quiet, silent state; if pressured to respond or act, there can only be a helpless shrug, 'Oh, what's the use'. Let's look at some specific examples.

Faced with *real-world stress*, the individual becomes withdrawn and resigned. He feels hopeless and powerless in the face of the overwhelming 'relevance' of others and the complete 'irrelevance' of his or her own presence. This feeling is actually 'unreal' and reveals, in fact, an inability to appraise self and self-worth.

Faced with *body stress*, the individual is genuinely unable to act to prevent the stress or discomfort worsening; his or her experiences do not account for self-care and protection. Whether they become ill or not depends purely on chance and the presence of others who can and do help. They begin, though, to exhaust their body's ability to override low-level problems.

Faced with *interpersonal stress* the individual becomes withdrawn and helpless and expresses this in relationships as a loss of stamina or fatigue. It is, in fact, a characteristic way of dealing with issues or demands with which the individual has no ability to cope. Tiredness becomes a structured way of withdrawing, used time and again to excuse inaction and unresponsiveness.

Adulthood   What has happened so far sets up the individual for what we earlier called *step 2 and 3* risks. The individual lives under routinely intense body states with poor body-mind integration. CNS and endocrine operations remain poorly co-ordinated and in a state of over-activity. At the same time, the growing realization of inadequacy leads to an increasing inability to act on this body-state pressure and a fatigued helpless posture is used both to avoid interpersonal challenge and to distance the mind from the internal body state. Lowered immunity and over-reactive CNS-endocrine responses become routine; a healthy, protective homeostasis — the normal, learned pattern of adult body-mind functioning — does not occur. Like all body activity, homeostasis and body-mind integration require proper learning, training and experience; the repression of emotion, the denial of the right for individual training/learning time result in a very fragile body-mind system.

Thus we find our cancer-prone person as he or she faces adulthood. What stands between him or her and the presence of cancer? Two factors. First, if she or he can avoid excessive exposure to carcinogens, the cancer-risk remains only a risk. Secondly, the kind of relationships the individual enters into as an adult can literally make or break the cancer-predisposing pattern. The human personality and, to a degree, the body systems are remarkably malleable. It is quite possible for an adult of twenty-one to meet someone who completely changes his or her life: the person may be exposed to an intimacy and a caring that can effectively restore a twenty-year-old pattern of unhealthy functioning to health. It really is never too late to make major changes in personality and body functioning.

Three basic types of relationships are relevant to our cancer model.

i *The status-quo maintaining relationship* This kind of relationship can best be described as purely a 'holding' or superficial one in the sense of it not actually affecting the cancer-prone person in any fundamental way. Unfortunately what happens to cancer-prone people quite often is that their unemotionalism and avoidance of emotional challenges ensures that they marry or live with people who also want a bland, unemotional life. The cancer person then simply continues as before, slightly more socially secure for being married, but not changed essentially in psychology, behaviour and habits. These people live together, often evolve a comfortable, supportive

existence and basically carry on the pattern of the cancer
person's home life. The isolation, loneliness and inattention to
self remain present, but become even more ignored; 'being
married' is a favourite cliché used to cloak real problems inside
oneself. Since the person is not 'alone' and goes through the
motions of being 'happily married', there appears to be nothing
wrong. Once the cancer-prone person is comfortably settled in
this kind of relationship, and once there is regular exposure to
the actions of carcinogens, cancer is an inevitable development
of the patterns learned at home. Adulthood and subsequent
relationships will offer no hope or assistance. This is the
hypothetical worst situation; all the necessary factors are
present and it is only a matter of time.

ii *The supportive relationship*   In these relationships you
are fortunate enough to meet and relate to someone who actually
pressures you in one way or another to change or modify your
habits. I call it the good-mother or good-father relationship; your
partner, usually just through instinct or commonsense, sees
what you need and gives it to you. You are looked after; your
partner will actually take the time to see that you start doing the
right things for yourself. This isn't necessarily a conscious effort
on his or her part; he or she simply takes over in certain key
basic respects. Often it is at a very simple level, to ensure you eat
better, or bath more often, or brush your teeth, or rest occasionally, or rest when you're sick, or otherwise make you feel more
secure. These simple changes in habits can be enough to hold
your cancer-proneness at bay. Your partner might keep an eye
on your drinking, your smoking, your weight, might make sure
you get enough exercise, and so on, all of which act as checks on
habits learnt at home.

     If you welcome this intervention, you will actually modify
your body systems sufficiently to stay cancer-free. If however,
as some people do, you fight this intervention by, for instance,
continuing to smoke when you have been told to stop, then
you're playing a dangerous game with your potential for cancer;
make this a routine and you'll be in trouble. We'll look at these
reactions closer in the next chapter.

     Relationships like these can help you to survive for years,

but there is one key flaw in their constitution. If you lose this relationship, or if it is put at risk, you lose your protective regulator; if you have not learned to take responsibility for looking after yourself, have not actually used the relationship to develop as an independent person (and therefore as a body-mind entity), your dependency on your partner leaves you vulnerable to anything that changes it. Say he or she goes off with someone else, falls ill, needs looking after him or herself, or dies, and you cannot keep up the regulation, then you risk cancer starting. I feel sure this pattern of regulating within-a-supportive relationship accounts for the presence of unexpected cancers in people who die from other causes; the cancer was there but remained contained. It also helps to account for dormant cancers which suddenly erupt following changes in the regulatory pattern; and it also, I believe, accounts in part for the fluctuations many cancer victims experience when a known cancer suddenly flares up after years of apparent recovery.

iii *The radical relationship*   This kind of relationship is the life-changing type in which the person's entire structure of thinking, feeling and body-mind patterning changes for the better. The relationship, in fact, need not necessarily be supportive in the sense described in (ii) above although this helps the transition in the early phases. However, it must be penetrating. In these relationships the partner pushes through the cancer-prone individual's blandness and avoidance of emotion so that the *real* state of helplessness and body stress can be exposed and dealt with. This usually means that the cancer-prone person becomes deeply upset, regresses and has to learn a new constructive way of being upset; it's like being made to grow up all over again, but this time getting it right. Great patience, love and skill are needed, but they ensure that the cancer person's body-functioning changes in a healthy direction and, moreover, that this change occurs so fundamentally that even loss of the relationship does not deprive the individual of the change. (We'll look at this later.)

   If you are lucky enough to experience this kind of relationship, you will almost certainly radically alter your cancer risk. It is a method incidentally that I hope will become available in the future as psychologists, psychiatrists and other professionals uncover more about relationships and how valuable they can be. Therapeutic efforts would naturally take longer than a radical relationship to achieve beneficial effects. On the other hand seeing a skilled therapist may start you on the road to putting your own relationship right a lot quicker than you could do on your own.

FINAL WORD

The information above completes the overall framework. We have identified the basic factors necessary for cancer to occur, the three levels of behaviour that generate the habits which create the cancer-forming conditions. We have spelt out the psychological and interpersonal contexts in which these habits are most likely to occur. And lastly, we have drawn a psychological profile of the high risk case, the worst-possible case. All the psychological and behavioural habits have to be present to create the right body-states for cancer cells to survive. It is not strictly a psychological model but a psycho-biological one. Think of it in a straightforward way, in terms of the simple day-to-day habits that you are taught or which you create. If you can recognize your pattern, link it to your daily life and *then* do something about it, there's no need for you to get cancer. As in one of those science fiction space games, a set of conditions has to be met before anything happens; spot the pattern, make the changes and avert danger. Even minimal changes in your living habits or the way you think can help you.

In Chapter 4 we'll see how the model applies in some of the more common cancers, then in Chapters 5 and 6 I'll give you much more advice on how to prevent cancer, or how to modify your life to fight cancer if you've got it. Remember, cancer is a psycho-biological event with horrendous organic consequences, but the first step in helping yourself and avoiding cancer is a mental one. The final controller of the body is your CNS. Use psychology, use your mind to make the changes. The first step is psychological, and is in your hands.

CHAPTER 4
The Psychology of the Common Cancers

So far we've looked at how the cancer model operates in a general fashion. We need now to examine the more commonly-found cancers and to link our model to them. This will help spell out in more detail how the process of getting cancer works, thus enabling us to look at how to avoid cancer. In this Chapter we will examine lung cancer, breast cancer, cancers of the digestive system (bowel, intestines and stomach), cancers of the reproductive system (cervix and penis), and skin cancer.

Before we examine each type of cancer we need to introduce two concepts about body function to guide us in our exploration. We need to know how to think about healthy body activity in general, and how to think about healthy activity in specific areas or organs of the body.

HEALTHY BODY FUNCTION

Most of us are taught that a healthy body is one in which every part of the body does what it's supposed to do. We usually conceive of this in a fundamental way; the heart beats and pumps blood into the arteries, its job is to pump. The digestive system digests and absorbs food and its job is to allow the protein, fats and so on to pass into the body while eliminating waste. The lungs take in oxygen and expel carbon dioxide; their job is to purify the blood. So long as they *do* the job, according to this formula, then the body is healthy.

Now, while this is true in a practical sense, it does not adequately define a *healthy* body; this simply defines a *functioning* body. Think of an uncared-for engine in an old car; it still turns over and moves the vehicle, but we'd hardly call it healthy — just functional. Think of an old car with a meticulously looked-after engine, serviced regularly, and so on — that engine would be called healthy. The first engine could pack up at any time; the second we could trust to go on for years. It is this sense of healthy functioning that will concern us most in what follows.

As the body is a remarkably resilient entity we can get by, i.e. go on living, even though we might be overweight, smoke and drink too much and don't exercise. We therefore make the assumption that everything's all right. The problem is that just surviving isn't suitable as a model for healthy functioning. Four elements are required before we can say a body is healthy. First the *function* of each part must occur much as we defined above, i.e. each organ and body system must do its job. Second, each part must be *used* fully, i.e. exercised or worked, preferably regularly. Third, the organ or body system must be *rested* and allowed to *recover* after activity. Fourth, the organ or body system must do its job in the *context* of *real-life activity*, i.e. it has to function well when operating in concert with all other organs. It has, as a matter of course, to take its place in the body-mind *team* that we define as the individual.

This model of healthy functioning is, of course, something which not all of us achieve, but it is a very useful way to think about the body and what the body is used for.

HEALTHY FUNCTIONING IN INDIVIDUAL ORGANS

Much the same model can be applied to any individual organ.

We can think, for example, of a genuinely healthy heart as being one that pumps blood around the body, is regularly exercised to its full capacity, is allowed time for rest and recuperation, and lastly works well in conjunction with other organs, as a member of a well-drilled team.

You can imagine what would happen if a particular organ, while healthy in every respect, couldn't work as part of the team. Imagine what happens, for example, if you suddenly have to run in an emergency: your heart pumps hard and your central nervous and endocrine systems send out the alert signals. But what happens if your lungs, your stomach or your intestines aren't working well at that particular moment? If you have a cold, or a bronchial infection your lungs can't cope with the demands of running and you'd be forced to stop. Say you've just over-eaten, your stomach can't cope and you get cramp or you vomit. Again you'll have to stop. One could argue that these are unusual coincidences, instances of unfortunate sequences of events, but many people, whether through chronic smoking, over-eating, or some other excess, routinely are not able to operate their body systems as a team. Hence the importance of thinking about healthy functioning in the more complex way we have identified here. Now let's get on to the common cancers. Keep this view of the healthy body in mind as we go along.

THE COMMON CANCERS

Lung cancer   Strictly speaking, lung cancer is any one of a number of cancers found in the respiratory system of the body. Anywhere along the route from nose and mouth to lungs, cancer can develop. So one can get cancer of the mouth, nasal passages, sinuses, throat, larynx, windpipe, and so on. Most common though, is cancer of the lung and the usual site for the cancer to develop is in the bronchi, that part of the lung where oxygen from air breathed is absorbed through fine membranes into the blood. The classic symptoms of lung cancer — developing an unexpected cough or a change occurring in an existing cough with spitting blood, breathlessness and variable pain — are all caused by the tumour obstructing the action of the bronchi and slowly destroying the lung.

Our bodies survive because we breathe — an activity we never cease to perform as long as we live. Much of the lung's activity is automatic; the central nervous system regulates our breathing through hundreds of electrical links which synchronize and pattern the muscles and other components needed for the lungs' activity. However, within this automatic framework the individual still has considerable power to interfere with or override the pattern or synchronicity of breathing. We can, for example, hold our breath for short periods. We can breath shallowly or deeply according to our choice. We can also interfere with what actually goes into our lungs; we can inhale a wide range of things from clean air to smoke and fumes.

Above all, through gradual exposure, we can condition the lungs to accept levels of functioning in which the lungs operate *automatically* at levels well below their capability and below what is healthy. The obvious example is smoking tobacco. Over time we can condition our lungs to operate with high levels of tobacco smoke in the air coming into them.

But there are other ways we can 'set' our lungs at specific, reduced levels of functioning. We can, for instance, avoid exercise — not just in the sense of never playing a sport, but by avoiding ordinary taxing things like walking up steps. The result is that the lungs never draw deep breaths. We can also restrict our lungs' functioning by cramping our chest muscles; chronically shy, nervous or tense people, for example, have very poor breathing habits which do not permit muscle expansion and force the lungs to breathe under both tension (fear) and a reduced level of efficiency. As a last example, we can cramp our lungs by not shouting or not crying when everything inside us is geared to expressive lung action, such as when we're angry or upset.

To sum up, we can interfere with the healthy function of the lungs in two basic ways:

i Through what we breathe.
ii Through how we limit the action of our lungs.

If we go back to our cancer-creating framework, you'll appreciate that both of these forms of interference fit comfortably into the model.

Step 1: Exposure to carcinogens　　To start the cancer chain moving requires exposure to carcinogens and the most common carcinogen for the lungs is tobacco smoke. To qualify as an *exposure* risk, i.e. *step 1* risk, you need to engage in smoking in a fairly specific way. You have to use smoking habitually as a means of coping and to have reached the point where it has become an end in itself.

What we breathe in　　Many people, particularly partners of smokers, are exposed to secondary smoke inhalation; they live with smokers and can absorb tobacco smoke in just the same way as smokers do. It doesn't have to be tobacco smoke; exposure on a routine level to fumes, to anything harmful inhaled, puts you at an *exposure* risk. You get psychologically used to the exposure, or feel you have no choice, and you start the process of accustomising your lungs to operating at a reduced level.

No matter whether you're a smoker or not, a heavy smoker or a light one, if you have allowed your lungs to become conditioned to accepting a reduced level of clean air on a daily basis consider yourself at step 1. I suspect that this might go for virtually any kind of pollution and not necessarily tobacco smoke; tobacco smoke has become such a big issue simply because it's the one we are most exposed to. If, however, your job or hobby involves you in close contact with any irritant you should still be wary.

A second point arises here. We can all tolerate some carcinogens in our lungs and cope with quite consistent exposure to poor air even on a routine basis. If, however, this is balanced by periods of cleaning the lungs out on an equally routine basis, risks are reduced. High risks are incurred when episodes of cleaning out are almost non-existent; an omission which is commoner than you might think. All too often the act of getting proper air into your lungs is left till last.

How we breathe　　As vast publicity has been given to smoking as a cause of lung cancer, it has been easy for people to lose sight of the fact that how a person breathes also plays a part in exposing him or her to carcinogens in say, tobacco smoke. Expose a healthy, fully functioning and robust lung to a daily input of tobacco smoke and the chances are the lung will cope well. Reduce the efficiency and robustness of the lung (without reducing the amount of smoke) and you increase the risks of the carcinogens overwhelming the natural activity of the lung. For a less than efficient lung then, less exposure to carcinogens is required. Again, it's easy to arrive at this state of affairs; don't exercise, don't stretch your lungs, don't use them to shout or to cry when you need to. Even athletes, if they stop training, quickly reduce the efficiency of their lungs.

Don't think that because you don't smoke you're free of risk. Your individual habits, your personal relationships (living with a smoker for example) can make you vulnerable – sometimes more so than a smoker. The risks are created by a combination of what you allow yourself to breathe in and how you actually use or exercise your lungs.

Step 2:Overriding the body's normal response   Ordinarily the body would respond quite promptly to over-indulgence or to inefficiency in the lungs. No one likes to wheeze at the slightest exertion or to breathe fumes in endlessly. The body has to be taught to accept these levels of functioning. As outlined in the last chapter, you can condition the lungs to accept low levels of discomfort by using higher systems like the CNS to override the lower signals of discomfort. Anxiety in a social situation, indeed anxiety or insecurity in any situation, creates an intense and urgent focus of attention which easily overwhelms most lower signals. Continued or repeated experiences set up a patterned avoidance of lower signs amounting in time to a kind of body blind spot; the mind eventually learns to ignore input from the area — the lungs. This pattern then becomes incorporated into anxiety-coping styles of behaviour used by the individual and the risk established.

So much for theory. How does this work in practice? Well, as you're growing up and beginning to cope with adulthood and all its anxieties it matters far more to you that you cope with the burden of inadequacy and lack of confidence you feel inside than that you take good care of your lungs. Most of us have to go through this and there is a time in everyone's life where being accepted and being regarded as part of a group matters more than anything else. The idea that growing up is a fun, anxiety-free experience is purely for the story books. Real life is troubling and real people use whatever socially-approved crutches are available to get by. Currently it's smoking, which unfortunately puts the lungs under considerable stress, a fact that most of us would readily admit to if we were being frank. However, this merely keys us to the fact that young adults have vulnerable lungs; how can the individual make it worse?

Easy. Smoke to ease the feeling of being anxious. Then make it a blind spot; smoke without thinking, use smoking to cover the fact that you're anxious. Key the act of smoking to every moment of even vague anxiety and pretty soon it will have become so well-established that you won't even remember that there was a time you experienced signals of discomfort.

More, the experience of smoking becomes an act of personality expression, a statement about who and what you are. I'm reminded of several people I know who smoke under what I can only regard as combat conditions for their bodies; one chap insists on smoking when he's working on his car. There he is, sweating under the weight of spare parts, his lungs straining under the normal exertion of intense body activity and the double load of the cigarette he's smoking at the same time. But for him it's all part of his image: he would never think of doing the job without the cigarette in his mouth. I know other smokers, people who smoke more than he does but whose pattern of actual smoking is quite different: they are what I consider to be sensible smokers. They smoke, certainly, even inhale. But the moment the act of smoking is inappropriate, they stop. Thus, if they have a game of tennis to play, or if they have to be fit for something, or if they have a cold or sore throat, the first thing they do is stop smoking. This gives their bodies a chance to cope better. Their heavy smoking is broken up and interspersed with episodes of healthy breathing. And in this time, they re-establish contact with their body signals and in particular with what's going on in their lungs. They are still at risk, true, but less so than my mechanic friend who isn't such a heavy smoker but smokes at the very time when every instinct in his body is shouting for him not to.

When this kind of override pattern gets established we can be sure that deeper issues within the individual's personality have helped to make the habit of override persist.

Don't get the impression that this is a simple, wilful act only performed by peculiar kinds of people. It is very easy to grow up in our culture and to smoke — a potentially self-destructive act — for quite healthy psychological reasons. I'm thinking here of smoking as an act of rebellion or assertion of individuality, in particular the role it plays for women seeking to break free from the stereotyping of traditionalist societies. One female smoker I know in Athens put it this way:

> 'In Greece women have few avenues to express their independence. It took me five years to smoke openly and several more before my family tolerated it. My smoking is my independence. When you ask me to give it up you don't know how much of me I would have to destroy. I need it everyday, not because I like it, but because every time I smoke I break the mould of how my society thinks I, a woman, should behave.'

Having lived in a few traditionalist societies I can only add that the above statement does not exaggerate the pressures placed on many individuals. In these circumstances it would be psychologically unhealthy to 'back down'. I feel sure that elements of this feeling also enter into the smoking habits of many women in more industrialized societies. For them, the kind of risks I've been discussing here are secondary to the assertion of independence. Understandable and in need of sympathetic attention, but as you can see, further evidence of how easy it is to get yourself exposed to the dangers of habitual override of body signals.

The point of all this is that given exposure to, say, cigarette smoke as outlined in step 1 above and habits as described in this section on override will both intensify the exposure to potential carcinogens and ensure that the local signals of distress in the lungs, throat and mouth remain unattended to. In time therefore, local cell damage will occur in these areas. The area affected would then have to cope with the damage without assistance from the main body systems and at the same time would be under repeated exposure to the very agent doing the damage in the first place — certainly a no-win situation if ever there was one.

Step 3: Lung cancer and lowered immunity   To ensure that *cancer growth* itself takes place, our bodies' immune system must fail to cope with the neoplastic growth which results from the exposure and vulnerability that occurs in *steps 1 and 2*. Much of what was described about the way people can lower immunity in the last chapter applies here, but we can be more specific and describe the kinds of habits that can lead to a lowered resistance in the lungs.

For healthy functioning, the lungs need exercise. You need to exert them in good clean fresh air. The lungs also need to rest in clean, comfortable conditions. Above all, you need to use them as part of normal, daily living. It is essential, for example, to lose your temper, raise your voice, or at least *say* something when you're angry. All your other body systems are geared to it and failing to express the emotion shuts off a vital part of the body's outlet. You block the team-work right where it matters most. A cancer-prone person at risk from steps 1 and 2 can prevent cancer forming if they are able regularly and routinely to use the lungs whether they are crying, running, making love, working or relaxing; these activities will help ensure that the immune system is working properly.

Few people realize how large a part the lungs play in the body's healthy survival. It isn't just a matter of breathing. Talking, eating and moving all involve the lungs. When you don't feel happy you tend to cut down on these activities; you eat less, communicate less, exercise less, and so on. All have their effects on the efficiency of the lungs, which is why colds and other respiratory illnesses so commonly occur at a time of low psychological ebb. You quite simply let your lungs run down and, feeling miserable, you avoid taking simple caring steps like getting out of a draught or not getting wet.

I am here reminded of a case I saw of a non-smoking woman who used to work in a smoke-filled kitchen, ironing away day in and day out, coughing, sweating and really placing her lungs under pressure. She developed lung cancer; her husband who sat smoking in the kitchen was a very heavy smoker, but he was careful to get plenty of fresh air and not smoke if *he* had anything physically demanding to do. It was a consideration that saved his life.

Was it the exposure to smoke that did the damage to his wife? Well, ultimately, yes, but it was the matrix of factors starting with the personal difficulties between them that inhibited her from saying anything about his smoking (and his lack of sensitivity) that really counted. Her inability to act and her willingness to subvert her body symptoms to her desire to maintain the family peace did the damage. She overrode her body signals.

In another case I knew in Africa, an underground worker who lost a lung through lung cancer was renowned, prior to getting cancer, for his lack of commonsense while working. Angry and frustrated with life for many reasons, he routinely ignored safety regulations and the need to take proper rest breaks; he would virtually force himself to work to exhaustion in stifling heat and dust. Remarkably few of his colleagues developed lung cancer simply because they never took the personal risks he did. And, surprisingly, many of them smoked while he was a non-smoker.

In both these cases the personalities of the victims could be described as manifesting a kind of angry helplessness. The woman in the kitchen was always at the doctor with chest problems and he had tried to point out to her the dangers of letting herself get run down. But she was determined to carry on expressing, we felt, her basic attitude to life — a profoundly fatalistic one. The underground worker seemed determined to make life as difficult for himself as possible, carrying the same disregard for his body everywhere he went; he drove badly, drank too much and eventually succumbed to an overdose of drugs and home-made beer at the age of thirty-seven. Significantly, he died alone. In all the time he lived life so aggressively, he shared his emotions with no one, played no sport and did no exercise.

These two examples of step 3 risk show how non-smokers with

deficient immune systems allow themselves to become at risk from cancer by *exposure* to carcinogens and by *overriding* their body symptoms of distress. Take away either of the latter and you'd be left with the immune risk, which need not have been serious.

The psychology of lung cancer   The trouble is that really high-risk people tend to evolve an overriding psychological pattern which helps to ensure that all the bad breathing habits listed above become a routine part of their lives. They smoke or expose themselves to carcinogens, they override all body-stress symptoms in their lungs, they continue their habits when their bodies are taxed, and they allow their immune systems to run down as a matter of course. Why? Let me introduce you to a case study.

Burt, a forty-eight-year-old businessman, had lung cancer. Reared in a comfortable middle-class home, he had married fairly young, done well in his job and was generally regarded as a success in both his personal and business lives. However, talking to Burt and his wife, it was possible to identify the psychological patterns that had led to Burt gradually exposing himself to cancer risk from his early twenties onwards.

As a youngster in his family, Burt had been a model child — thoughtful, hard-working, and 'very little trouble', as he put it. In fact, he had been encouraged by his parents to 'cope' from an early age; not for him tears and emotions like other children — he was, rather, the strong silent type. This characteristic had attracted Pam, his wife; it had helped her later to account for the fact that in their married life, Burt was a removed, even distant person. 'Not in any obvious, unkind way,' she reported, 'but he doesn't show much. He doesn't argue, get upset, or even express an opinion much. He's closed. And yet I sense so much is going on inside him. So much pressure.' In fact, this was absolutely true; Burt was under pressure and his only outlet was smoking. He had started smoking in his teens and had used it ever since as practically his only means of expressing what was going on inside him. Studying his smoking habits was remarkably illuminating about Burt; what emerged was at complete variance with the picture everyone had of him.

Starting first thing in the morning, Burt would get up, stretch and yawn in front of an open window while inhaling deeply on a cigarette. Throughout the day, no matter what was happening, Burt had a cigarette in his mouth: at breakfast with the kids, in the car, at meetings, on the golf course, everywhere. What was even more interesting was the way Burt used his smoking. When he was calm, it was slow and unhurried; like a cowboy playing with a gun, he toyed with the smoke, caressed the cigarette, inhaled and played with the feelings as he finished the cigarette to the last shred of tobacco. When he was upset, the cigarette became a symbol of the pressure he was feeling inside. He used it to reassure himself, looking at the cigarette for long moments as a means of taking his mind off what was worrying him. He used it to break his nervousness, smoking in short puffs, finishing one cigarette half way and lighting another, all while appearing calm and relaxed on the outside. 'Are you nervous?' I'd ask. 'Oh no, I'm never nervous. I'm just thinking, that's all.'

When Burt was angry, the cigarette became a weapon. If I asked him something he didn't want to talk about, he'd look at me with a bland expression on his face, take a deep breath and envelop me in a cloud of smoke. Immediately I reacted, he quickly apologized and made a joke of it, but it was no joke. When Burt was angry with himself, his breathing and smoking became painful to watch; he would inhale ridiculously deeply, contort in discomfort, cough and then draw again until there were tears in his eyes. And he never stopped, even when he began to develop chronic bronchitis.

You can see the pattern. Burt lived through his smoking. He ensured that his lungs were massively and routinely exposed to a carcinogen, he systematically overrode his body signs of stress and he forced his body to perform routinely under what I thought were almost combat conditions. He's the only person I know who played golf while smoking and yet inevitably won. That's how hard he drove his body. And he became a local 'character' as a result, which automatically ensured that he had to play with a cigarette in his mouth, even if he hadn't wanted to.

All this was damaging enough, but in addition, Burt had a

characteristic 'helplessness' pattern when it came to interpersonal relationships and coping with most stresses. Unable to
attend to his own body needs, or to express any emotions he
might feel, he resorted to a kind of hollow 'conformity'. He said
and did all the right things but one felt he never actually took
part or did things spontaneously for himself or reacted as an
individual. He simply went on smoking and waited for someone
else or circumstances to solve the problem. 'Emotionally, he
waits until you get over it,' said his wife, when asked about how
he coped with upsets in the family. 'In reality,' she said, 'he is
quite manipulative in a passive, non-verbal way; he puts
pressure on us to get back to normal as quickly as possible.'

In fact, Burt was a highly dependent person even though
he gave the opposite impression; most of his success and coping
arose through simply conforming or performing as he was
directed to. Faced with anything out of the ordinary — a
business reversal or an accident to a child — he became helpless,
almost paralyzed. Later, when his wife had an affair with
someone else and threatened to leave him, Burt finally gave in,
felt incredibly sorry for himself, got depressed and lost interest
in everything. It was during this stressful interpersonal episode
that he developed the cancer. I felt sure it had been waiting for
his general immune system to fail; when his wife had finally
threatened to leave, she removed her support and Burt's
systems collapsed.

Much of the psychological research on lung cancer has
found a similar pattern of psychological functioning. Lung
cancer victims, for example, have been found to be unemotional,
to deny internal or indeed any problems, to be highly dependent
on others and socially highly conforming. And it is these
patterns that shape the behaviour we know is needed to start
cancer. It is a vicious chain reaction: such an individual doesn't
express emotions, denies the need to be upset, then over-
indulges in a convenient and socially acceptable form of
expressing stress like smoking, drinking, poor eating habits or
fast driving until it becomes a fixation. Their insecurity, their
unwillingness to make fools of themselves, to be seen as 'weak',
and the tendency to feel helpless leads them to avoid being upset
or stressed, which in turn leads them to avoid using their bodies

properly. These factors, combined with the use of a carcinogen, eventually lead up to the development of cancer.

The point here is that, again, we must try to see lung cancer as arising out of a series of steps. Burt was an extreme case; other people might share many of the psychological and behavioural characteristics that Burt had, but without the chain being completed, the risks drop.

I hope you can see now that getting lung cancer involves a relatively complex chain of events, so it is not enough to think that you can avoid it by not smoking. Apart from the fact that some lung cancers are not caused by tobacco smoke, as we've seen, living with a smoker can be risky if you have vulnerabilities in the areas we've described. In our society we ought to concentrate on minimizing the presence of carcinogens and irritants like tobacco in public (and private) places, even more than simply condemning smoking. If people want to smoke, fair enough, but let's be sure they don't inflict their smoke on anyone else, possibly less capable than they are of coping with it.

Stomach, intestinal and bowel cancers   After lung cancer in men and breast cancer in women, stomach cancer is the next most prevalent form of cancer. Taken together, stomach and bowel cancers are the commonest forms of cancer affecting both men and women alike. The stomach and bowel are concerned with two vital activities in the digestion and absorption of food into the body; digestion takes place mainly in the stomach, absorption in the intestines. We can term this area the digestive tract and think of the cancers to be found there as cancers of this tract, sometimes also called the *alimentary* cancers.

The stomach's function is to take the chewed-up food we eat, which arrives in large, non-absorbable chunks, and by mixing it with gastric juices, reduce it down to smaller molecules. The stomach looks like a smallish, expandable balloon with strong muscles surrounding it which contract in waves (the peristaltic movement) to propel food down into the intestines where the bulk of the absorption takes place. The inner lining of the stomach is made up of thousands of little glands that secrete the gastric juices and hydrochloric acid needed to dissolve the food. At the exit from the stomach is a muscle which acts like a trap door (the pyloric sphincter), balancing the peristaltic movement and holding the food in the stomach long enough for it to be digested. The stomach does not digest carbohydrates (starch and sugar), but it does digest protein and some fats.

The intestines are responsible for much of the absorption process; there, food is further reduced into simple compounds (mainly simple sugars, or glucose) which pass through the intestinal mucosa (the lining of the intestines) into the blood and lymph systems. The intestines are responsible for breaking down carbohydrates and fats and for their absorption along with water and electrolyte salts. Fats and carbohydrates are used by the body for energy, while protein, as amino acid, is the building block for body cells and structures. The bowel, with its bacteria, is the receptacle for all waste products which are expelled eventually through the anus. Two sphincter muscles control the exit of waste from the bowel, one on the inside and one on the outside. These stay shut until ordered by the central nervous system to open.

Altogether the digestive tract is an extremely important part of our body. Where can it go wrong, or more pertinently, where can we make it go wrong? There are a number of considerations. First, we may eat or drink materials that the digestive system can't handle properly. Secondly, we may eat or drink too much and overload the system. Third, we can affect the rate of secretion of gastric juices and acid – we can over- or under-secrete – and cause imbalances of the enzymes, and so on, involved in the process of digestion. Fourth, we can interfere with the actions of the muscles, especially the pyloric muscle at the exit from the stomach and the anal sphincter muscle in the bowel. This traps food in the stomach or intestines for too long or too short a time. Fifth, we can interfere with the rate of absorption from the intestines; hormones play a central role in regulating the rate of carbohydrate absorption, for example. The hormone, insulin, keeps the absorption rate low, but stress produces adencorticosteroids which speed it up. You thus can overload or underload the energy levels in the body.

Cancers in the stomach tend to form in the middle or lower end of the organ, either as swelling or projections into the fluid, or as spreading ulcers. They do their damage by bleeding and ulcerating, blocking the movement of food or destroying the lining of the stomach and eventually the stomach wall. Outside the stomach, tumours tend to form in the large intestine and bowel (rarely in the small intestine) and originate in the cells of the glands directly in contact with the food.

Symptoms vary from individual to individual, but inevitably involve indigestion, distended stomach and discomfort in the abdomen. As the tumour grows, pain begins. In stomach cancer you begin to lose your appetite, lose weight, and sometimes develop anaemia from loss of blood through ulceration. In intestine-bowel cancers there would be an unexpected change for the worse in bowel habits; you might suddenly become constipated for no apparent reason, or have periods of constipation alternating with diarrhoea.

To sum up, our habits or behaviours interfere with the functioning of these organs in two basic ways:

i By what we put in, i.e. what we eat and drink and in what quantities.
ii By how we interfere with the jobs these organs are supposed to perform.

Let's now use our model to examine the links between these two voluntary levels of interference and the development of cancer.

Step 1: Exposing the digestive tract to carcinogens   We are concerned in *step 1* with the process of exposure to carcinogens and, just as with tobacco smoke and lung cancer, clearly what we eat can contain carcinogens which may set up the digestive tract for cancer. It has not been as easy to identify specific carcinogens in the diet as it has been to link lung cancer to tobacco smoke. However, we can infer from much of the research that has been done that at least some of the material we eat or drink does contain carcinogens and that some can become carcinogenic in specific internal contexts, such as an over-acidic stomach.
What we eat   Earlier this century stomach cancer was

the major cancer killer, found very much more frequently among working-class people than upper-class people. Today stomach cancer is occurring less and less frequently especially in Western, industrialized societies where standards of food production have steadily become more rigorous. The obvious conclusion must be that poorly preserved food and un-hygienic eating conditions exposed many people to contaminated or infected food which in turn resulted in stomach cancer.

The point is that, even without being certain which foods contain carcinogens, it is entirely possible that eating foods in specific ways may set people up for a *step 1* risk. If we don't cook our food, or preserve it properly, we risk chronic gastritis or inflammation of the intestines, both of which have been linked to cancer. Leaving certain other foods out of diets, too, can predispose people to gastric cancer. In South America, for example, eating food high in nitrates (which means low consumption of green vegetables) has been linked to cancer. Other research has similarly linked lack of fibre or bulk in diets to bowel cancer. The same is true of diets with too high a fat content.

From our point of view, therefore, we would expect a certain kind of eating preference to be linked to *step 1* risk. Many of us have intense likes and dislikes about what we eat; numerous adults still preserve a childhood dislike for cabbage, or some other once-detested vegetable. Persistently avoiding eating greens, for instance, seems likely to put you at risk. There are also many people who, as a matter of compulsive routine, avoid both vegetables and high-bulk food and instead consume great quantities of fried or fatty dishes. Habits like these may expose individuals to the same kind of risk that tobacco smoke does. Most of us are familiar with the situation where a chronically unhealthy diet is stuck to obsessively, even aggressively, and used way beyond the catalytic effect that eating should have. Eating 'what I bloody well like' can be as satisfying emotionally, as anxiety-relieving, relaxing and nerve-steadying as any cigarette.

How we pass food through the system   There is a second way that we can become exposed to carcinogens — we can keep food in the system longer than we should. Consider a common instance: you eat a meal, but due to anxiety or some other disturbance, you don't relax the muscle releasing food from the stomach. You are so tense you 'freeze' everything below the waist. Now if this goes on for long enough, two things can happen: you leave the partially digested food in your stomach, giving any carcinogens present double the time to go to work on the ducts in the stomach walls, and secondly, if you cannot relax the pyloric muscle properly, the food has to squeeze past, scraping and irritating the area immediately before the muscle. Any carcinogens present in the food are again given the opportunity to react with a vulnerable area of the organ. Significantly, most cancer tumours do occur in this area of the stomach.

Another instance concerns the operation of the anal sphincter muscle. After eating, digestion and absorption have been completed, the muscles in the anus will (or should) open and allow the waste out. If you are chronically constipated you risk leaving the waste in the bowel (and then backing up into the intestine) for a long time. Again, any carcinogens present can cause trouble; moreover, like the action of the pyloric muscle in the stomach, if the muscles can't fully release, the ensuing friction and pressure cause irritation, tearing and inflammation, creating vulnerability in the organ.

Imagine, therefore, what happens if you (a) eat an unhealthy diet and (b) can't operate the major control muscles properly. Think of the effect of this as a chronic habit on the digestive tract. The key word here is *chronic*. If this only occasionally happens to you and if you have good periods where everything operates normally, then all should be well.

Step 2: How we interfere with the normal digestive functions
Clearly any damage done in *step 1* can be quite serious, but I am convinced that on their own these acts will not actually generate cancer. To do that further action is needed on top of a *step 1* habit.

Once we have eaten something and it is in the stomach, we can interfere with it in a number of ways. We can produce an imbalanced set of secretions in the stomach that can create an environment harmful to the lining of the walls. We can secrete too much acid through the ducts (as people who get ulcers are presumed to do). We can also secrete inadequate levels of gastric enzymes, thus reducing the efficiency of the digestion of protein. Excessive anxiety over a long period of time is known to affect stomach function and the consequences of indigestion, cramps and sluggish digestion are familiar to all of us. Imagine what happens when these occur on a daily basis. These 'interferences' are nearly always produced by CNS and/or endocrine involvement with the lower systems.

Again, *overriding* is a feature of behaviour at this level. For some people, eating in company (perhaps with the family) can be an ordeal with a lot of anxiety attached to it. It is an easy matter to override symptoms of body discomfort while focusing on the tensions around the table, as many anorexics know. Too-rapid eating, gulping food down without it being chewed, forcing the food through the body all have their effect on disrupting the activity of the stomach and intestines. The formality and tension traditionally attached to Japanese meals may well contribute as much to the high rate of stomach cancer in Japan as highly-salted or smoked food. And let's not forget that anger and many other emotions can easily accompany eating behaviour; swallowing angrily, refusing specific foods to make a point against someone can all, when chronically practised, have a serious effect on the process of digestion.

The same goes for the absorption process. Chronic tension and chronic anxiety can mean that the process of absorption in the intestines becomes inefficient with the result that too little raw material passes into the body.

Step 3: How we live, lowered immunity and its effects on digestion   One of the problems with having poor digestion is that it interferes with daily life. Having to spend hours on the toilet every day trying to empty your bowels for example, having full, distended intestines, or having stomach cramps and other pain, not only result in abnormal levels of digestion and absorption, but also tend to reduce your general level of body and mind activity. Lack of energy and irritability can keep you from getting enough physical exercise, for example. Pain or discomfort can interfere, too, with other activities, like making love. And it can create or foster depression and general emotional

lethargy. Having a vital part of your body operating in a reduced
or vulnerable way creates problems for the body-mind team;
your immune system in particular requires adequate and
regular supplies of nutrients and protein. Without being able to
rely on these, you get a patchy, irregular or reduced level of
general body surveillance. Again a vicious circle is easily begun
in which digestive problems slowly condition the other body
systems to operate inadequately.

Take being constipated. The one thing that helps your
parasympathetic system relax (the sub-system of the CNS
system that controls the sphincters), is if you can take your
mind off it and let the system work without mental interference.
One way of doing this is to exercise, but you won't want to
exercise if you're in pain or discomfort. And so the cycle builds;
you don't exercise, you can't take your mind off it, you become
obsessed with it and neglect other aspects of your body and their
demands.

The psychology of digestive tract cancers   The really high-
risk person practises habits which ensure that all three risk
conditions are met: excessive exposure to carcinogens, interference in digestive, absorbative or eliminative functions, and a
general reduced level of immunity and body co-ordination act
together to create cancer. There is a psychological pattern
associated with this cluster of habits, structurally very similar to
that described in Burt's case earlier.

Fundamentally, the pattern of habits related to these
cancers appears to be laid down far earlier in life than in some
other cancers. You learn eating and toilet habits in the family,
and once they've been instilled they may well not change for the
rest of your life. Thus we can envisage a child growing up to
attain *steps 1 and 2* risks quite easily. A lot of people favour
specific kinds of food, and many people experience, and even
expect, constipation or indigestion as a routine part of their lives,
without doing much about it. So, in what circumstances are the
three steps cemented together? A case study will help us to
understand the circumstances better.

Carole was a married woman in her mid-thirties who
developed a bowel cancer, and was operated on successfully by
re-section. Interviewed about her life and habits before cancer

developed, she revealed what I think is a typical psychological background. Coming from a home with very serious and very religious parents, Carole always remembered associating pain and anxiety with her bowel movements.

'We were a strict household. Everything had to be done on time; you weren't allowed to be an individual or a nuisance. I got by most of the time, but one thing I couldn't do was go to the toilet efficiently. I used to sit there, conscious in our silent house of how long I was being. I imagined my father looking at his watch and saying to mother, "What's keeping her?". Everything was done to a schedule. If you broke the pattern you were immediately questioned as to why. All very tense-making.'

As a teenager, Carole began to avoid using the toilet at home, preferring to wait until she was at school or in a public place. By then it had become an almost overriding obsession. Her parents discouraged open shows of upset and it is clear that, as she had got older, Carole was expressing all her pent-up distress through her chronic constipation. She survived as long as she did by using laxatives extensively and by the fact that she was a very attractive, caring person.

When she married (at nineteen) and was, in her words, 'free of home at last', unfortunately she gradually entrenched her patterns in the wrong way. Instead of using her new-found freedom to do something constructive about her habits she built her and her husband's emotional life around them. Apparently in retaliation for her having to escape from home to go to the toilet, she now made her husband tolerate hours discussing, focusing and helping her constipation. They 'lived' around her constipation. If she'd managed to evacuate her bowels, the household was happy; they made love (otherwise it was too uncomfortable), went out to dinner, dancing, and so on. If not, which was most of the time, an 'air of despair' (her husband's words) settled over everything. Everything centred on the problem; books were read, doctors consulted, remedies tried. All other life ceased, going out became impossible, and being essentially a gentle and quiet couple, they maintained this pattern for years.

This is a pretty clear example of how the cancer cycle builds up in a high-risk case. Please remember that all three steps have to be linked. It is no good thinking you will get cancer if you are constipated, or if you won't eat greens, or have cramps at meals. You have to *fixate* on the problems, do nothing realistic about them, express your anxieties through them *solely* before you can be sure of running a high risk of getting cancer. Carole, like Burt, had begun to live through her problem. If she became upset, angry, or distressed, the first thing to suffer was her bowel action. Her husband confided to me that when she was upset with him her constipation got worse. At those times, laxatives just didn't work. Asked if she expressed anger, or upset in any other way at all, he said, 'No. Overall it's all that matters. If she's unconstipated she's happy; if not she's down. No in-between.'

A note on cancer and body fixations   This is a good time to raise a very important point. In both Carole's and Burt's cases their habits had become fixations, in fact, their sole fixations. This is, I believe, the essential *psychological* pattern that we must look for in someone at risk from cancer. The habits they develop converge on one basic act of behaviour — smoking, eating, constipation or whatever – and they literally *live* through those habits; that is, their emotional lives are expressed almost exclusively through smoking or whether or not they're going to the toilet, and so on.

If you were able to spread your emotional or stress-coping habits beyond *one* organ or *one* set of behaviours, it would help to break the fixation on a single habit. Nowhere does this issue surface more clearly than in the research on ulcerative colitis and cancer, and nowhere in the medical literature is there such an interesting instance of what I'm describing.

Ulcerative colitis is a fairly common condition. It has as its chief symptom chronic inflammation of the colon or bowel (as does a very similar condition, Crohn's disease). About a third of all people with this illness go on to develop cancer in the same areas. What is significant about this condition which, incidentally has no known cause and is thought to be related to psychological stress, is that when compared with other people, individuals with ulcerative colitis or Crohn's disease, tend not to smoke. Further, it seems that on average few smokers get inflammatory bowel disease. Now this as-yet unexplained anomaly seems to me to be a clear case of what I've outlined in this chapter: if you focus on a single habit of coping with nervous tension then it is more damaging to your system than if you can diversify your habits of coping and thus relieve the pressure on one specific area. In fact, just this approach has been suggested for ulcerative colitis victims as a means of alleviating their symptoms and (presumably) of lowering their risks of later getting cancer. They have been encouraged by some experts to smoke in order to do this. Certainly, from my own experience in doing psychotherapy and behaviour therapy with ulcerative colitis sufferers, a key element in successfuly reducing their symptoms is to teach them better means of coping with stress. The best results were obtained if they were introduced to something quick, basic and easy to do in order to help them stop using their bowels as a focus of immediate attention. Often something fundamental like smoking, tearing up a book, crying or just phoning a friend worked well.

Once this had been established I could then build better, more thorough-going behaviours that in time would encourage my patients to develop better organ-use and better body-mind integration.

The key individual psychological characteristic to look for is the obsessive fixation on *one organ* of the body. When this occurs in the absence of any other significant form of coping with stress or expressing emotion, the pattern is set. Let me repeat: in my opinion, unless new behaviours are learned, there is little hope that the pressure on the specific organ will be eased. The psychological pattern that Carole exhibited helped to ensure that the bad habit she learned as a child never changed for the better as she grew up. Further, the kind of relationships she entered into were not strong enough to break her obsession, thus providing the final link in a long chain.

Breast Cancer   Cancers of the digestive tract and cancers of the respiratory system are, in a sense, easier to comprehend than breast cancer. At least we can envisage the cause-and-effect relationship involved in lung cancer quite clearly; you smoke, which pours a carcinogen into your lung which, along with all the other factors we have discussed, does the damage. Similarly we can easily picture carcinogens in food or drink setting up a vulnerable stomach for cancer. But what can one make of cancer of the breast? How can it be possible for a physical agent, like tobacco or food, to get in there in the first place to start the damage?

Let's begin to answer these questions by getting a clear picture of what the breast actually is because while a great deal has been written about breasts (and, in particular, female breasts), very few attempts have been made to place them in what I think is their proper psychological and sociological context. Similarly much has been written about breast cancer, but practically nothing on the psychological reference of the organs themselves.

What is a breast? We can answer this in a number of ways. *Physiologically* the breast is situated on the chest in males and females and comprises a nipple which is the access point (where contact with the outside world begins) and the focus of sets of glandular cells (alveoli) arranged in circular fashion around the nipple. These cells are capable of secreting milk, which passes through tiny ducts to microscopic openings in the nipple. The whole system is drained and protected by an interconnected lymph network – part of the body's immune system. This network is linked, in turn, to major lymph nodes under the armpits.

Surrounding these lobes of alveoli and further supporting and protecting them is a varying quantity of fat. The quantity of this fat dictates the size and shape of the breast we see externally.

Developmentally the breasts undergo considerable change in females as they grow older. Male breasts can, of course, change too; masses of fat can be added, for instance, to give (almost) the appearance of adult female breasts. The use of hormones (as in transvestism and transsexualism) can also develop the male breasts very similarly to a woman's. The changes in female breasts usually start in adolescence when, due to growth hormonal secretion, the breasts enlarge gradually to their adult size. A further change takes place, too, in pregnancy when the alveoli fill with milk produced by prolactin (another hormone), ready to breastfeed the baby. A final change takes place from middle to old age (though not in every woman) when the breasts may shrink and appear withered.

So what is the *function* of the breast? In men it is nothing so important as in women, but they have, nevertheless, a cultural and sexual role to play in the sense of having neural sensitivity and being a measure of physical attractiveness; a well-developed chest with little or no breast growth is considered attractive, excessive breast growth is judged unattractive. In women the breast has two distinct functions. At a basic anatomical level, the breast exists to feed the baby after birth. Culturally, the female breast has more complex status. In Western society, and in Western-orientated cultures throughout the world, it is perhaps the part of the female anatomy most frequently used as a fetish; that is, as a marker-of-sex, a fraction of the whole person used as a symbol of sexual status. In the popular imagination, heavily backed up by advertising and the entertainment industry, the female breast serves both as a means of identification and, given the presence of other fetishes (pretty face, hair) as a sign of sexual attractiveness or appeal. In consequence breasts play an important role in the emotional and psychological development of most Western females; from puberty onwards the shape and size (or lack of it) determine to a surprising extent whether or not a woman feels she can be 'identified' as a woman. For many women breast development is a reassuring activity, giving them a form of social security. For some women, too, this fixation can play an important part in the shaping of their personality and interpersonal relationships. An important second corollary of this cultural focusing on breasts is the role played by breasts in sexual behaviour; after kissing, fondling them is the commonest step in the development of sexual intimacy.

In other cultures female breasts have a different status. In Japan, for example, breasts were not traditionally as much a fetish as other anatomical features: indeed they were often tightly bound to minimise their presence, and much greater emphasis was placed on overall body movements, including voice, fragility, submission, and so on. In some traditional African tribes buttocks assume the status given to breasts in the

West, with the role of breasts in cultural and sexual activity being strictly confined to their baby-feeding function.

So, quite a complex picture. What does this mean for us here? Let's define breasts in terms of how they are *used* in Western society (where, incidentally, the bulk of breast cancer cases are to be found in the world), and in particular how an individual woman is liable to use them.

From adolescence onwards women are conditioned to fixate on breasts as one of a number of fetishistic signs of both sexual and personal worth. The breasts may be examined and caressed, prodded and pinched on a regular basis — by the woman herself as much as by an admiring partner. Equally, they can be ignored, — not just in a casual way as we might ignore the third toe along on a foot, but in an attempt to deny their presence or their significance.

Breasts can be used as a form of communication to men, as well as a sign of superiority or inferiority to other women. In sexual intimacy the breasts can be used in many ways: caressed, bitten, squashed, pulled or sucked, all as an integral part of love play.

Lastly, breasts are used in and beyond pregnancy where they are again manipulated, touched and sucked by the nursing baby. This formulation permits us to identify the following ways a woman can affect her breasts:

- By actively manipulating them or letting someone else manipulate them, i.e. letting them be felt, squeezed, etc.
- By actively ignoring them and not looking after them.
- By failing to secrete appropriate hormonal instructions to the breasts, and thus hindering their normal development or function.

Breast cancer nearly always occurs in the cells lining the ducts (the alveoli) supplying milk to the nipple. From there it grows into a tumour (felt as a lump) which in time can become attached to the muscles beneath the breast or to the fatty protective skin above them. Metastases (secondary deposits) form in the lymph nodes under the arms, travelling to them via the lymph drainage network in the breast.

It takes quite a long time for the cancer to be felt even as a tiny lump. Early symptoms of breast cancer are minimal; sometimes an eczema-like condition on the nipples appears before a lump is detected, but this is rare. A lump doesn't necessarily indicate cancer either; it can be a form of fibroadenoma (a benign tumour) or simply a local thickening of fatty tissue. Nor is pain a clue; cancerous lumps are rarely painful.

Breast cancer is essentially a Western-society disease; it is practically absent in the Far East and in many parts of South America. In the UK and US, by contrast breast cancer is increasing in incidence. It is also found more often in middle and upper class women and less frequently among lower classes.

Let's now return to those earlier questions and see how our model accounts for this form of cancer.

Steps 1 and 2: Exposing the breast to risk   Breasts don't get exposed to smoke or other carcinogens, so how can they be said to be exposed to risk? Some researchers feel that what we eat can ensure certain carcinogens are absorbed into the body. One of the arguments offered to account for the difference between Western and Eastern breast cancer rates suggests that it is due to differences in diets, that the more refined Western diet somehow exposes women to breast cancer. No identifiable carcinogen, however, has been found and in lists of statistics which show people as running a low breast cancer risk, diet doesn't figure; having a first baby under the age of twenty, being of low social class, having many children, or having one's ovaries removed before the age of thirty-seven are all found to help women avoid breast cancer, but rarely, it seems, what they eat.

If, however, we examine this list a little closer, we can identify two possible ways of introducing a form of carcinogen into the breasts or rather creating a condition whose effects will be very similar to having a carcinogen present. (That is, if we define a carcinogen as an irritant.) At the same time we can also try to link dietary and cultural patterns to these sources.

Hormones and the breast   You'll notice from the list that most items focus on hormonal influences. Pregnancy is a major hormonal event in the body; having a pregnancy tends, as it were, to wipe the slate clean hormonally. It doesn't matter

how their owner felt about the breasts before – the effects of
falling pregnant force the breasts into basic baby-supporting
activity. Similarly, having a pregnancy before the age of twenty
is most likely to force hormonal-breast behaviour patterns into a
relatively healthy adult mode of functioning and replace any
cancer-risk activity present beforehand. Having multiple pregnancies has the same effect; moreover, in this instance there
isn't much time to re-impose bad habits or create pathological
patterns. Interestingly enough, early and multiple pregnancies
are very much more common among poorer people, which may
well account for the appearance of this social class on the low-
risk list.

What does this all mean? To my mind the reason that pregnancy seems to protect against breast cancer has to do with the fact
the pre-existing body-mind framework is *overridden* by a whole
sequence of body events which impose an organization and order
on mind-body networks. Pregnancy is one of the few events in
life in which this occurs; nature, if you like, takes the body in
hand for nine months and dictates a set of habits, endocrine
secretions, and so on, over which the higher centres have
relatively little control. Pregnancy radically alters the body-
mind networks and the new, learned patterns tend to persist
thereafter. Having a baby acts as a kind of organizer; emotionally, psychologically and somatically, the breasts are never the
same again afterwards.

If pregnancy is nature's restorative it suggests that
hormonal influences are present in breast cancer and points us
in the direction of a possible habit, or set of habits, that could
predispose a person to cancer risk at the first and second levels.
During pregnancy the breasts grow and fill up, accompanied by
two supporting systems: first, endocrine centres high up in the
brain secrete a hormone that tells the breast to grow and secrete
milk. It is a simple, overpowering message that the breasts are
well-equipped to deal with. More important though, the psychological and cultural state of the pregnant woman is geared to
acting in support and close integration with these hormonal
messages, and the growth of the breast. Not only is the breast
physically better supported with special brassieres during pregnancy, but the mother, and those around her, focus attention,

time and consideration on them in a completely new asexual way. Pain, or discomfort, for example, are now attended to and the mother regards her breasts as a healthier, more integrated part of herself. The breasts never know a better time; perfect co-ordination with psychological states (culturally the sex-identity pressure is off), endocrine states (hormones) and proper care and maintenance.

Now compare this state with another fairly common but very different state. You're in a relationship in which you're insecure, not sure of yourself or your partner. During your love play you become tense or apprehensive; you can't relax, are not aroused, don't feel safe, and yet you're behaving as if you're taking part. Your partner begins to feel your breasts. Perhaps he does it too roughly, so that you feel uncomfortable or even in pain. Let's stop there. I can't think of a more 'out-of-synch' state to impose on the breasts; you're not aroused, therefore you're not secreting the hormone pattern that usually accompanies the activity of making love. You may even be secreting stress hormone which will prepare your body and its organs for a fear pattern — not the relaxing rhythmic set you'd need for climaxing. At the same time, your breasts are being manipulated *as if* their internal state was in line with the manipulation. Your muscles are not relaxed properly and above all you're not reacting or receiving the appropriate feedback from your breasts (arousal) which completes the feedback loop needed for full love-making. Last, you daren't stop or complain because it might break his rhythm, upset him, creating more anxiety for you than it's worth. So you override the discomfort, and all the body signs that should warn you to stop and worse, you simulate spontaneous love-making activity. It's like jumping down from a wall and landing on your feet without bending your knees. I think you can see how this kind of situation, if repeated often enough, can set up a physical state inside the breast in which the wrong hormonal pattern is present, the correct pattern is absent or weak and the muscle cells and sense receptors are simultaneously subjected to inappropriate override and physical irritation, even pain. Blocked ducts, giving rise to swellings which we call cysts, may well be caused by one or more of these actions; for example, secretions in a duct can dry up or the duct become blocked. Significantly there is some evidence to suggest that having a history of cysts and/or benign tumours may predispose a person to eventually getting cancer.

This combination of neglect, override of discomfort, and subjecting the breasts to behaviour for which there is no internal (hormonal or muscle) 'keying' can I believe create a situation within the breast which is analogous to *steps 1 and 2* in, for example, lung cancer. The breasts are being forced to work, as it were, under pressure and in the presence of the wrong hormone. Poor team work again. Significantly another risk factor associated with breast cancer is having treatment for, say, mastitis, a non-cancerous breast disease, with androgens (the male hormone). This may again be a case of the wrong hormone being in the wrong place at the wrong time.

Diet and hormones   What we *eat* can interfere with the normal hormonal balance in the breast. Very interesting research from the University of Manchester has recently reported on the importance of sugar consumption in relation to breast cancer. Briefly, it suggests that eating a lot of sugar (as we do in the West) can interfere with the uptake of insulin in the body. Insulin is a vital hormone, and it may well be that too much sugar passing into the blood and cells interferes with, or at least alters, the ability of other hormones to complete their function. Interestingly enough, many of the breast cancer sufferers I've seen had something of a sweet tooth; several in particular harboured a passion for chocolate and ate it in large quantities.

I suspect though that if this dietary factor operates, it will do so in co-operation with other factors and not just along the lines of 'eating too much sugar gives you breast cancer'. My own hypothesis is that excessive sugar consumption is often to be found in people who use food (or rather, certain types of food) to alleviate anxiety. Cancer-prone people may add to their risks if they eat sweets excessively on a chronic basis and if they engage in the kind of override and hormone-imbalancing activity described earlier.

Step 3: Exposing the breast to cancer growths   The fact that the female breast is so closely protected by its lymph network should, in theory, ensure that growths are easily eliminated instead of spreading, as often as they do, to the armpits. The problem is that habitual inattention to the breasts in terms of examining them, caring for them properly and in responding to symptoms of discomfort and change can create problems for your body-support systems. If, emotionally, you don't 'want' breasts or try to ignore their existence, you can condition your central nervous system to ignore the input from its sense receptors in the breasts. It's as if you try not to have to attend to them. Do this as a routine and you seriously lower the ability of the immune system in the area to react properly. If, further, your immunity is generally at a low level then you add to the risk.

The psychology of breast cancer   While little has been written about the predisposing behavioural and physiological states, a great deal has been published about the personality of the breast cancer victim. In fact, it is one of the better-researched areas in that the main finding — the failure to express anger or negative emotions openly — has been relatively well-established.

Other traits have also been reported in breast cancer victims; some researchers, for example, have commented on the general inaccessability of their breast cancer victims, suggesting that they hold people 'at a distance' in relationships. A number of psychodynamic-orientated writers have suggested that breast cancer victims have a poor sense of their identity as females and consequently 'repress' their feminine sexual feelings and characteristics. Others have found subjects to be excessively altruistic (putting others before self or putting ideologies before feelings) and tending to be family-bound. Most researchers of whatever persuasion would agree though that in principle, the lack of emotional outlet for internally-felt anger and distress is the single most important characteristic.

The problem with much of this research lies in its generality. Some of the terms employed in articles (altruistic, asexual, denial of femininity, etc.) are not, I feel, clearly enough related to the basic structure of behaviour we are considering. It is more revealing to examine the abstract traits as they occur in the context of an actual case study.

Let me describe the case of someone I was fortunate to know well *before* she developed breast cancer. Marie was the thirty-two-year-old wife of one of my patients. In explaining what happened to her I hope you'll be able to grasp the complex interaction between the social and psychological worlds in which she lived and the kinds of habits I described earlier which put her at risk from breast cancer.

Marie had married Henry, my patient, at the age of twenty-six and I got to know her, not in order to help her, but my patient. I asked to see her to help me fathom what was going on in his life. In fact her husband, a professional man in his late thirties, was not a seriously disturbed person at all; he had difficulty in relaxing and coping with the ups and downs of his job, but over the time I saw him and his wife, separate and intriguing patterns of problems emerged concerning her.

Marie was the eldest daughter of a country farmer and had grown up in relative isolation under what I eventually realized was a crippling set of psychological circumstances. Her younger brother had been something of a troublesome presence as they grew up and much of Marie's time at home had been spent in coping with both his crises (he later became psychotic and was hospitalized) and her parents' distress at what was happening to him.

At the age of twenty-two Marie had finally left home, much to her parents' anguish. She left the country and worked abroad for several years before returning and quickly marrying Henry. She had in fact felt very guilty about 'deserting Mum and Dad' as she put it, but she felt that if she didn't get away she would suffocate. She had had few friends, had kept very much to herself and, in fact, was an extremely responsible and hard-working person. Abroad she'd held quite senior positions at the companies she's worked for. She'd had few relationships and, I suspect, had married Henry (a childhood friend) to avoid becoming involved with her family again.

Throughout her time abroad and during her married life she has maintained contact with her family and asked to see me (after one or two routine sessions about Henry) mainly to help her cope with her family life. Not, note, with her husband's problems. Thus for nearly three years before she developed cancer, I got to know her, her life with her husband, her life at work and, above all, her relationships within her family. Let me tell you about them in sequence and you'll see how her psychological existence helped to shape her habits.

At *home* she'd grown up to be the first person to whom her parents turned in helping them cope with her brother. Her own growth and development had been neglected in order to support and comfort her parents and to explain what was happening to her brother. If he was in trouble, it was Marie who talked to him or saw the doctors. She was regarded at home as the strong, independent one and was rarely given much in the way of attention or consideration. Not, I must stress, that she realized this at the time; she felt sorry for her parents, found them sweet, helpless and bewildered people. Deprived of the time to cope with her own problems, not given room to express feelings or to demand attention, she had, as it were, 'ceased to function'. Later, in discussions with me, she was able to identify the unexpressed pent-up frustration she felt towards her parents, her anger at being used and her intense sadness at their state and, latterly, her own. In quiet moments she realized how empty her life had been, how all the developments and excitement of adolescence had passed by in a blur of helpless frustration. Effectively she had not been an adolescent, had not experienced sexual explorations or intellectual challenge. They had simply not occurred because always at the forefront of her mind had been her anxiety and concern for her brother and parents.

In her *working life*, Marie had found at last the relief from pressure she'd always needed. But at the age of twenty-two, she'd had no experience of adult life and while abroad had focused entirely either on her work or occasional phone calls from home. She came home because she felt lonely and isolated abroad and had worried continuously about what was happening to her family.

In her *marriage*, Marie had very soon fallen into an old and familiar pattern. Henry was a pleasant, sensible man, although with many inadequacies in his interpersonal abilities, who as a result was very demanding. Soon Marie's life became what I thought was a living hell — split between being phoned daily by mother to cope with family crises and having to spend hours soothing and looking after Henry. When I began to see Marie I sensed an enormous distress inside her despite her assurances that she was happily married and had everything to live for. In time I became convinced that she was near breaking point; she was neglected and she knew it, but had nothing and no one to help her express her anguish. Her intense hopelessness was compounded, I think, by her realization that somewhere she had simply exchanged one set of demands for another.

Investigating her relationship with Henry, it became clear that she was essentially passive in their intimate side. Occasionally she had complained that he hurt her in their love-making, but she was reluctant to go into details.

Suffice it to say that the pattern of over-concern and over-focusing on others (being the 'powerful' one in the relationship with her parents and with her husband), which she'd learned at home were transferred first to her employer, then to her husband. And when I say 'over-focus', I mean it; Marie spent virtually every minute of her day thinking about Henry, worrying about him and planning for him. Thus, a quiet evening at home would be broken up by Henry's becoming upset with the neighbours; an evening out would be made tense for her by his dislike of the food. Just like at home; if there was something wrong, Marie took the responsibility, not because it was her fault, but that she felt she was expected to put it right.

Marie was long-suffering and exhausted. She had no time to herself, didn't know how to be 'selfish' or to focus on herself and, literally, was slowly becoming very run-down. She was psychologically starved of time.

When she developed a lump in her breast I saw her prior to her biopsy and a few more details emerged: initially she was very shocked, of course, but it soon became clear that her breasts (unbeknown to Henry, or me or anyone) had gradually become the focus of a great deal of hostility. Distressed about the lump she gave vent to a tirade against her sex, against her role and her body; she had always hated her breasts, didn't know what they were for, had ignored them, didn't see what men saw in them and complained that all they'd ever given her was pain and discomfort. She was clearly venting all her anxiety and fear on her breasts, but at the same time too she was revealing things about her attitude to herself. It seems that she could accept everything else about her body but not her breasts; they 'bulged out' she said and she couldn't pretend to be a 'nothing' — the characteristic way she tried to cope with everything. She also said that she liked sex but for one thing — her breasts: 'If only Henry would leave them out we'd be OK.'

While this was a distressing outburst for her I doubt it may simply have been precipitated by the discovery of the lump. Later when cancer was diagnosed and the lump removed, we had the chance to explore her feelings about herself more deeply and it became very clear that at a low level of consciousness she had systematically tried to pretend that her breasts were *not* part of her body. They had in fact always been a fixation for her and her own distress (and self-disgust at letting people use her).

Luckily with insight things improved for Marie in her relationship with Henry and when later she became pregnant, her doctors felt she was no longer at risk.

The point about this case is that I feel it presents the general pattern of habits in their real-life context: the avoidance of proper care and attention to a vital organ (the breasts); the override of discomfort and pain; the avoidance of proper teamwork and experience in love-making and, lastly, the general exhaustion and body-mind fatigue that lowers immunity. I must also point out that I believe it is wrong to characterize breast cancer victims as anti-sexual or even anti-emotional; all the feelings are there, but with little knowledge of how to act on them. When Marie finally did learn how to be more 'selfish' as she put it, Henry and her family could not compete against the weight of her own feelings. And indeed, she felt that her creativity and insight into people increased appreciably too. Freed of the obsessive focusing on single individuals, Marie was able to alter the structure of her personality that had previously all been organized around living for someone else. By altering the set of psychological links that had cemented her habits into a narrow unhealthy band of functioning, she was able to change her internal body-mind structures. It was a hard job and certainly Henry was never the same again, but I believe Marie will survive.

OTHER COMMON CANCERS

The cancers we've discussed so far in this chapter account by
far for the biggest part of cancer deaths; nearly sixty per cent of
all cancers in men and women fall into one of these three organ
areas. The other common cancers, reproductive organ cancers
and skin cancer account for much of the balance. Space does not
permit me to go into these in detail but I do want to raise a
number of points about each.

Cancers of the reproductive system   In women a
number of cancers can arise in the reproductive area. Most
frequent is cancer of the cervix with cancers of the ovary, uterus,
vulva and vagina being other, rarer cancer sites. Men can suffer
from cancer of the testicle, penis and prostate gland.

Like lung cancer, we can readily appreciate the fact that
these cancers occur where contact is made with material
entering from the outside world. Cervical cancer for example has
been linked to frequency of intercourse with different men, the
implication being that this in some way introduces carcinogenic
material into the vagina and beyond: inflammation and possible
viral infection then follow. However, we must take care in
applying our model to be quite clear what the psychological and
behavioural preconditions are in these cases. I believe a great
deal of unnecessary psychological harm has occurred to sufferers with cervical cancer by the sometimes uncritical publicity
these findings have attracted.

Cervical cancer   This cancer arises in the cells of the
membrane separating the cervix (the mouth of the womb) from
the vagina. It starts off as a tumour or an ulcer and can gradually spread into the uterus, vagina and the pelvic area. Symptoms are few in the early stages; later bleeding and an unpleasant vaginal discharge may appear.

Research has established an interesting set of findings
about this cancer. The actual carcinogenic agent may well be a
virus and much has been made of the role played in setting the
organ up for *step 1* risk by genital infections such as herpes
simplex and venereal disease. However, the condition has been

found to be present in lower socio-economic groups in most countries studied with the exception of those countries or communities where sexual activity is limited and/or personal genital hygiene is culturally focused upon. Thus nuns, Jewish and Muslim communities have low rates. It is four times more likely in prostitutes and in the wives of men who travel or stay away from home for long periods. As we noted in earlier chapters, cervical cancer is on the increase and is gradually becoming less limited to lower socio-economic groups in the West. The change in sexual morality over the last three decades is often cited as a possible cause in this respect. Let's apply our model.

Step 1 risk   It is not yet known precisely what kind of virus causes cervical cancer. However surveys have shown that the more promiscuous a woman is, the more likely she is to develop cancer in the genital regions. Research has also shown that the younger a woman is when she starts having intercourse, the more likely she is later to develop cancer. This appears to be especially true if she starts in her early adolescence.

These findings have to be interpreted with great care because of the sensitive personal and moral issues involved. Obviously, at the simplest level, if you have a number of sexual partners you will expose yourself to a higher risk than someone who has only one partner. This is true of other diseases too; venereal diseases, infections, irritations and inflammations tend to go hand in hand with a high number of partners. Indiscriminate sexuality carries a greater risk; if you don't know the people you sleep with very well there is no way that you would know where they had been before you. Thus you could easily be exposed to a wide range of viral agents without being aware of it.

Women who do have a number of regular sexual partners but who know them well and are not promiscuous or indiscriminate are at less risk. They can however be vulnerable if any one of their partners suddenly changes his habits and does engage in indiscriminate sex.

Poor personal hygiene in either partner can also bring risks. Women or men who do not wash properly (or at all) after intercourse can develop infections in the genital regions. The risks increase if this neglect is of a chronic nature. Indiscriminate sexual habits plus lack of adequate personal hygiene are probably the two highest risk factors.

Cervical cancer does not strike only at women who have many lovers. At risk too are women whose partners engage in promiscuous or indiscriminate sex even if they themselves don't. I have seen a number of women who have developed cervical cancer but who have never in their lives slept with a man other than their husbands:

I was treating a wealthy businessman for a vague kind of depressive illness. He was not an especially communicative person and so I saw his wife once or twice to glean background information. Angela was a very conservative, Christian woman, tense and nervous but quite alert and rather sensitive — a different kettle of fish from her husband. About a year later I happened to bump into her in an outpatients' unit at a hospital and we chatted for a while. She had just been told that her cervical smear indicated that she had cancer. One of the first things she said to me was: 'But I don't understand; I've never slept with anyone other than my husband, and that only occasionally.' She'd been reading all she could about cervical cancer, including a magazine article linking cervical cancer to frequency of intercourse. I left her very troubled because of what I knew and what I couldn't tell her — that while she hadn't slept around, her husband certainly had. In fact he was obsessive about it; he travelled up-country a great deal and slept with anyone who took his fancy. Clearly, in my mind, my client's wife had exposed herself to *step 1* risk (infection) as a result of his activities. Therapeutic ethics forbade me to tell her or indeed anyone else but I did tell him and this shocked him enough to try to limit his promiscuity.

What made matters worse for her was that she had had no idea that her husband had been having indiscriminate affairs. While she knew there were difficulties in the marriage she and her doctors were quite unaware of his practices. I believe that this happens quite often; that a woman develops cervical cancer, is treated for it, makes a recovery and then life goes back to normal and after a time she again finds herself with cancer. Re-occurrences like this could be prevented in many cases if the woman's partner was told about the risks he may be exposing her to. I know it is a delicate matter, but it needs to be done. It also makes a lot of sense when you consider that cervical cancer is one of the cancers that is routinely and successfully treated without major surgery or indeed many of the debilitating side-effects of other cancer treatments.

Step 2 risk   We must be clear that the risk in *step 1*, of being 'infected', does not alone guarantee a cancer growth. In the case I described above and in similar cases, far more is involved. How a woman makes love, and how she feels about intercourse also play vital roles in setting up risks. Making love, for example, when you are not properly aroused, and not secreting vaginal fluids, being tense in your vaginal muscles or tense in your pelvis can predispose you to friction, tearing, irritation and inflammation internally which, given a *step 1* risk, can be dangerous. Couple this with an inability to express your discomfort or take adequate steps to look after yourself and the risks increase.

Here is an example. Several years ago I saw a young couple who had been referred to me for help with sexual difficulties. Generally speaking sexual difficulties in a relationship arise either out of the female partner's not being able to make love or to have an orgasm or the male partner's inability to maintain an erection or habitual premature ejaculation. In this case though both partners were able to perform all aspects of intercourse, they were in love and neither was involved in sexual relationships outside their own. Their problems arose because they could not agree about how often they should make love. He wanted intercourse every day, she only two or three times a week. On the face of it, compared to other couples I saw, they seemed to have very little to complain about.

However, investigating a little deeper soon revealed a situation that I believe was putting her at a step 2 risk. The real issue between the two of them was his conviction that he had a right to sex whenever he felt like it. For him this meant every day, irrespective of whatever else was going on. He also believed that women had the same right and that, if they were healthy and normal, they too would want to make love every day. He was convinced that his girlfriend was handicapped by her fairly strict upbringing and, in his words, he was freeing her from her past indoctrination by insisting on making love daily.

She in turn agreed with him. Or certainly she had done at the start of their relationship and certainly she said she did in front of him. When I saw her on her own, though, a different picture emerged. In the beginning of their relationship she had accepted his ideas but over time she began to feel more and more unprepared for daily intercourse. She found that it tired her and often interrupted other things she was doing. But the most exhausting thing was his insistence that she have an orgasm every time they make love. This, he said, was to make sure that she learnt to enjoy sex as much as he did. Because ordinarily she could orgasm she felt there was no way out for her but to conform. In the beginning this had been all right but soon she felt under so much pressure that making love had become something of a nightmare. She just couldn't keep up and to preserve the peace she had begun to fake her orgasm. He sensed this, and her tension and apprehension about making love, and this formed the basis of their arguments — he saying that she wasn't letting herself enjoy sex and that she was faking her orgasms, she denying both accusations.

Once she had told me the full story I could see how severe the problem was. I sympathized with her, undertook to explain her feelings to him and sent her to see a gynaecologist for a check up. However I hit an unexpected problem when I tried to put her problems to her partner. He listened patiently to what I had to say (and I also tried to tell him a little about female sexuality) but when I had finished he smiled at me and told me quite simply that I was wrong, that it was every woman's right to enjoy intercourse just as he did and, moreover, that I had made up everything I had to say about her not enjoying intercourse or faking her orgasms. When, puzzled, I turned to her for confirmation, she looked blankly at me and then calmly agreed with him and denied she had ever complained to me. I saw at once that she was frightened to stand up for herself in front of him. She had chosen to save the relationship at the cost of her own opinion and as it turned out, her own body. Obviously there were aspects to their relationship of which I was still not aware and so I had to let matters rest there.

They took their leave of me and I never saw them again. However the gynaecologist I had referred her to telephoned me about a week later to say that her cervical smear test was worrying and that he wanted to do a repeat of it because he suspected she was in a pre-cancerous stage. A month later he wrote me a note saying that he had contacted the couple again and asked for a re-test but the man had refused and got quite hostile with the doctor for suggesting that there was anything wrong with his girlfriend. Neither of us heard more about this case but we agreed that their love-making habits had more than likely put her at risk because of the way she was being forced to have intercourse in a state of tension and distress.

You can get some idea from this report how the risk patterns build up. The woman in the relationship described above was habitually exposing her genital organs to tremendous irritation, was chronically over-riding her own symptoms of distress and engaging in a behaviour in the most inappropriate of ways. Her body systems were adjusting to her discomfort and the inefficient functioning of her genital regions. We couldn't be sure in her case if she was in a pre-cancerous state or not (without the second test) but she was clearly at risk. Imagine if her partner suddenly decided that it was his right to sleep with other women. This would constitute step 1 and step 2 risks operating together; where exposure to carcinogenic agents (through sleeping around) is coupled with an organ being misused or otherwise rendered vulnerable.

Step 3 risk: The cancer-forming chain is completed if, in addition to the kind of risks described above, an individual has the habitual low level of immune functioning we defined earlier. This is probably best summarized as being a general apathy towards your body and its care. Among my patients I often noted a kind of resigned sadness and listlessness coupled with a sense of passive resentment. This said in effect: 'If no one else can be bothered to notice my needs and look after me, why should I?' There were complex psychological reasons why any given person should feel this but the net result in each case was a lowering of resistance and a gradual distancing of concern for any problems or discomforts that appeared anywhere in the

body. It is this attitude combined with the habitual exposure to
the first two risk steps that permits cancer to develop.

The psychology of cervical cancer   Not a great deal has been
written about the psychology of women suffering from cervical
cancer but in my experience several crucial factors appear to be
present in high-risk women.

The first concerns sexuality. Paradoxically, most of the
women I have seen with this form of cancer had quite ambiva-
lent attitudes towards making love. Many of them were very
experienced sexually and often had started making love early on
in their teens; by and large they saw themselves as knowing a lot
about sex and as being competent in love-making. However few
of them obtained much actual sexual pleasure from having
intercourse. It appeared to have become a habit rather like
brushing your teeth — something you do every day but don't
think too much about, nor wonder if you enjoy it for its
own sake. Sexual activity to my patients meant primarily a way
of satisfying their male partners, a way of keeping a certain kind
of contact open in the relationship. Many enjoyed this aspect of
intercourse — the warmth, caressing, body-contact — but their
own sexual needs seldom formed a part of the act. Nor were they
discussed with partners.

The second factor concerns loneliness. While few of my
cervical cancer patients described themselves as being lonely it
often struck me that they seemed to have a dread of ever being
left on their own, so much so that they seemed to fill their lives
with activities as if they were afraid to find themselves with time
on their hands. They seemed to be reluctant to spend time on
their own and above all to spend time reflecting about themselves and their lives. When they were forced to be thoughtful by
circumstances, they tended to feel depressed and miserable and
anxious about not getting on with other things; they didn't seem
to consider their own emotional states, their own private feelings
to be important. Most equated this state with being lonely and
preferred to be busy focusing on 'getting on with things'. Many
also remembered feeling lonely as adolescents, remembered not
liking the feeling and trying to avoid it.

The third factor, closely related to the above two, was the

excessive attention most of my patients focused on men — and in particular the man they were living with. This tendency to over-focus on the male in their lives at the expense of their own identities semed to have been laid down in their teens. Maureen, a thirty-seven year old woman who had successfully recovered from cervical cancer, tells a typical story:

'I started sleeping with my first boyfriend when I was thirteen. I didn't have a particularly happy home life, my parents were quite old when they had me and home was a pretty dull place. Having a boyfriend and making love meant the world to me at the time. It took me away from the dullness. It was exciting and I felt grown-up. Of course it was scary too but I looked older than my years and I was quite an actress too. Once I'd been with a man I couldn't live without one; I kept thinking of what it would be like to go back to that old humdrum life at home. I went from one man to another in my teens because somehow it never lasted — I think I was too immature. All I know is that I just had to have someone to sleep with at night and at one point I remember not caring who it was.

'When I eventually settled into a steady relationship I made the mistake of giving in to his every whim. I was so used to being seen as a sex object that I would worry if he didn't feel like making love. It had become a kind of drug; if we didn't make love I would suffer withdrawal symptoms and feel useless. It took me several relationships after that before I realized that sex isn't everything. Now I try to be more real and demanding in my relationships.'

To this day, though, Maureen struggles with her fixation on sex. She believes that if her partner wants to make love she must always be ready to do so no matter what her feelings are at the time. In other respects, in other parts of her life, she is healthy and self-protective. She has a good, responsible job for example, in which she more than holds her own with the men she comes across. She is a health-food freak and she jogs regularly. Her blind spot is her attitude to sex and to men and in this respect she has learnt to override her own needs systematically.

It was the combination of over-focusing on sexual intimacy as a measure of self-worth and on using sexual intercourse as a

means of getting security that most characterized the women I
saw with cervical cancer. Even Angela, who we met earlier, had
similar preoccupations. While she was never promiscuous (and
was put at risk by her husbands' affairs) she too was over-
focused on her sexual relationship with her husband. Her moods
were almost completely dictated by whether or not they made
love:

'When we make love I know that he loves me. I feel
fantastic and it will keep me happy for days at a time. I keep on
remembering it and it sort of fills me up, makes me feel like a
woman. I seem to get confident, cocky even. I walk in the street
glowing and triumphant. When I see other women, my friends,
who I know don't sleep with their husbands, I feel superior, as if
I'm on a different plane to them. But if he comes back from a
trip and doesn't want to make love (and we don't talk about
this, I just sense it from his mood) then it's as if my world
collapses. I watch him for the slightest hint of affection. I get
nervous and irritable. I don't go out, I don't want to see my
friends. I feel depressed, nothing matters any more.'

Angela never shared these thoughts with anyone, least of
all her husband and she firmly believed that all other women did
the same.

In sum then, like the lung cancer high-risk personality may
overfocus on smoking, the woman who is at high risk for cervical
cancer is liable to overfocus on sexuality and sexual intercourse.
This in turn seems to involve a neglect of other aspects of contact
and an over-dependence on males. Ultimately the woman learns to
neglect or ignore her own needs and habitually to disregard any
feelings of discomfort she might experience.

If we think about cervical cancer arising out of a complex
interaction of the factors discussed here it helps you form a
picture of where things go wrong. Again, the thing to watch for is
over-focusing on a single organ or a single action for the expression of a wide range of emotional experiences.

Cancers of the male reproductive organs   Although
the incidence of cancer in the male reproductive organs, in
particular testicular cancer, is reported to be on the increase,
little has been written about these cancers. Like the increased

incidence of genital cancers in women one suspects that changes in social attitudes have helped to create the climate for increased risk due to increased sexual contact. Poor personal hygiene is another factor to be considered, as too might be masturbatory habits. To illustrate the latter points I would like to describe a case of penile cancer in a young man whom I saw briefly. I would like, incidentally, to have written more about these cancers but this one case is the sum total of my experience in this area.

Mike was a twenty-eight-year old anthropology graduate who had spent a good deal of his life alone in Third World countries doing research and, as far as I could gather, thinking about nothing else but his penis. He was an extremely difficult person to help or indeed to glean information from but eventually he did reveal the following about his personal habits. From the age of thirteen he had masturbated every day and though he bathed when he was able to do so he had no notion of how to clean or care for his penis, felt guilty about sex and his penis, had no contact with women (except for once visiting a prostitute in Zaire), had little contact with his parents and even less with the people for whom he worked. From the age of nineteen onwards he had begun to have bouts of acute bladder infections which he had tried to ignore. Once he suffered a serious liver infection. It is my blief that his infections stemmed form the same origin: he was uncircumcized, he masturbated daily and did not know that the foreskin over the head of the penis has to be worked back and cleaned quite often. Without so doing, the head of the penis becomes a very unhealthy place indeed; in his case I felt sure his inadequate washing contributed to his penile cancer. Two other factors, I think, helped: his ability to ignore quite debilitating symptoms (and smells) without seeking advice and his habit of masturbating while wearing his trousers. He'd been told as a child never to touch his penis ('it was unclean') and his way of getting round this was to rub away at it through his trousers thus ensuring further inflammation and irritation through the material's contact with the skin and the presence of dirt and sweat from the material. Again, in the limited time I had with him, he presented fairly clear evidence for the model; three factors or sets of habits operating together to form cancer. Need-

less to say, I referred him to hospital where he appears to have
been cured by chemotherapy.

Skin cancer   This is a fairly common disorder and except
in a handful of rare cases, seldom serious in the sense of causing
death. It is commonest amongst fair-skinned people who have
undergone long exposure to the sun and it is on the increase,
significantly in white-skinned (as opposed to black or dark-
skinned) people and in areas of the world in which suntanning is
fashionable. In one study, for example, a definite correlation
between severe sunburn and the development of skin cancer has
been found. However, more than just exposure to sunlight is at
work. Here is an illustrative case in point.

   Two brothers, both farmers had worked for most of their
lives on the same farm and under the same conditions of
exposure to sunlight and yet only one developed a mild skin
cancer on his lip. Why? Well, I can't be absolutely sure but the
wife of the cancer-free farmer did remark to me that as far as
she was concerned her husband didn't get cancer because for
years she'd made him wear a protective lip cream despite his
protests and being mocked by his brother. I inquired further:
both found dry lips one of the worst features of working out in
the sun all day (they both wore hats — this was in the tropics).
The brother who developed cancer refused all remedies, laugh-
ing at his brother for wearing 'lip stick' — this was in the days
when males who used deodorant were regarded as 'queer' — and
proudly displayed his cracked and coarsened lips as proof of
how he could 'take it' in the sun. His personality differed
from his brother's, tending to disparage emotions; a quiet, silent
type, he seemed to burn inside with some unknown and
unexpressed anger. Here we have the necessary material for the
three key steps.

Step 1   You need excessive exposure to sunlight or heat, or
anything that will burn the skin.

Step 2   You need to avoid taking the necessary protection;
being exposed to sunlight, suntanning, even occasional burning,
are all relatively easy to cope with; when you routinely ignore

sensible precautions (and here I include properly exposing your skin to tanning) and/or override the pain and discomfort, then you're at risk.

Step 3   If, too, you fixate on this say, suntanning and have a lowered resistance, you've completed the cycle.

Again, note, it takes time and has to be a routine habit. Some of the psychological factors I've come across include: an excessive desire to have a tan; excessive avoidance of the sun; an excessive insensitivity to skin discomfort; and, lastly, a tendency to scratch or pick at sores and so on, on the skin. Underlying all four is usually an ill-defined anxiety and lack of adequate outlets for dealing with it.

SUMMING UP

What I have tried to do in this chapter is to take the most commonly-occurring cancers and see how the model I developed in chapter 3 applies to them. I hope you'll now have a better idea of how to think about cancer as a whole and are beginning to see how you could take steps to help yourself. Space unfortunately does not permit us to examine every cancer and of course there are some cancers to which this model may not be applicable. I am thinking, for instance, of some cancers that may be specifically genetic in origin (retinoblastoma) and others in which a known body weakness creates a cancer-like action as it progresses. There are some cancers, such as pancreatic cancer, which may well fit the model but owing to our present lack of accurate knowledge about the actual function of the organ, it is not yet possible to be certain. I have discussed the cancers where I think the model's applications are clear.

CHAPTER 5
Preventing Cancer

So far I've concentrated on examining how cancer is caused from the ground up, as it were, or more appropriately, from the body up. We've looked at how ordinary cells go through transitional stages before actually becoming cancerous and seen something of how the body's support systems interact with the basic cells to facilitate or retard the process. We've examined, too, the way an individual's habits of living interfere with the smooth operation of those systems — the central nervous, endocrine and immune systems — and we've put this complex interaction together in the cancer model developed in the last two chapters.

Throughout we've stressed the intricate interplay between body and mind trying to show that far from being unrelated they together form a deeply interacting single entity. Where we have examined the purely mental or psychological patterns associated with high-risk cancer people this has been clearly tied to the body-mind chain. When all three levels of risk occur in such an individual we can usually identify a common psychological (or personality) pattern linked to the high-risk occurrence. It has been stressed though that these psychological patterns have their effects by establishing the cancer-promoting habits in the following chain:

Psychological pattern	→	Habit patterns	→	Central nervous, Endocrine, and Immune system dysfunction	→	Cancer-forming process

It's not that the mind causes cancer, or that habits cause cancer, or that germs, foreign bodies or even carcinogens *cause* cancer; cancer requires the presence of sets of events occurring in a chain reaction.

Naturally, most people would prefer an either/or approach: cancer is either caused by the mind or it's not. And this tendency to seek straightforward cause-and-effect shows itself most clearly when the issue of how to prevent cancer arises. 'Stop smoking', 'stop eating junk foods', 'stop worrying' are some of the first convenient catch-phrases thrown up when anyone is asked to think about cancer prevention. In this book, though, I want to suggest that thinking about cancer prevention in a more thoroughgoing way as a body-mind issue can be just as 'simple' and yet provide individuals with a more accurate way of avoiding cancer. I shall argue, in fact, that it is eminently possible to use your mind to help avoid cancer. Not in the sense that a change in 'mind' or how an individual thinks will automatically or immediately free him or her from being at risk from cancer, but in the very practical sense that for most people the mind holds the key to unlocking the pattern of body-mind functioning.

Most of us have trouble in 'listening' to our bodies or in knowing what goes on inside, so to speak. There's so much else to focus on, so much outside us to think and worry about that we only really begin to take notice when our bodies break down and we can no longer take them for granted. Yet through developing the correct mental approach to our bodies it is possible to pick up body-stress signals far earlier than we do. Research has established, for example, that healthy individuals are far more aware of internal body events than unhealthy people and in experiments, perfectly ordinary people have been trained to develop a far greater sensitivity than they thought possible. Moreover people can be trained to change levels of body activity that were traditionally thought to be outside mental or voluntary control; for example, you can influence your heartrate, your skin sensitivity, your rate of gastric secretion, even the temperature in your hands and the electrical waves in your brain. Surprisingly many of these changes can be effected relatively easily; you can control your brain waves by simply thinking nice or relaxing thoughts and most people can be very quickly taught how to change heartrate and gastric secretion by altering thought and breathing patterns. Imagine how much more could be achieved if you were systematically able to retrain the way your body-mind systems functioned. This can be done by involving thinking, feeling and behaviour; it's harder than learning relaxation, but it is quite possible.

At this juncture I want to introduce to you a new concept of prevention. I want to suggest that if you're willing to devote the necessary time and energy to the task, you could use your mind to make changes in your behaviour that would effectively reduce any cancer-prone tendency you might have. I don't just mean 'stop smoking' or 'give up sweets' or 'start watching your skin for changes in moles.' Those are important pieces of advice, but they refer only to one level of risk, while cancer is a complex illness requiring sets of events to coincide in order to develop. Adequate prevention requires that you conceive of how to avoid cancer rather more thoroughly. It is possible to stop smoking and still develop cancer; a mole can change and it may have nothing to do with cancer.

Instead, I want to suggest that changing how to think about cancer and how to think about body-mind patterns can lead to changes in the habits that lead to cancer. If you want to think of cancer in a fatalistic 'you-either-get-it-or-you-don't' way, then so be it. If you want to have a fresh and thorough-going look at yourself with a view to understanding cancer, understanding where you contribute to your risks and doing something practical about it, then we're in business.

SOME PRELIMINARY WARNINGS

This chapter is largely directed at people who haven't yet developed cancer, and who want to be sure they stay cancer-free. Part of what I have to say is relevant for cancer sufferers, but more follows about them in the next chapter. Be warned, though, that some recommendations in this chapter are not appropriate for cancer sufferers. Evaluate what I have to say carefully in the context of your own problems, and discuss them with your doctor first if you do already have cancer. Remember, try to focus on *the gist* of what I am saying and try not to hang on to clichés or directives as if they were '*the* answer'.

Don't expect simple solutions. Most people welcome simple solutions because of their appeal: do *x* and all will be well; stop smoking, stop drinking, take laetrile, take exercise, take vitamin C. Thinking about cancer solutions purely on this basis is I think naive; far more is involved. In fact, assuming you do not have severely congested lungs or are dying of a heart condition, my advice would be *don't* stop smoking immediately, *don't*, in fact, give anything up straight away. Stop and *think* about yourself first. Be sure you're pointing in the right direction *before* you start changing, otherwise you could do more harm than good. Take time to understand things better first.

Try and be honest with yourself. If you can't, ask family or friends to help you do this. Someone somewhere will give you the clues you need. Remember, being bland about cancer or having a devil-may-care attitude to it and to yourself is no protection.

Getting started   Let me recap. We have looked at sets of bad habits, ways an individual has of routinely managing his or her body that result in the three cancer risk stages being present. We have described habits which ensure exposure of specific organs of the body to carcinogens (*step 1*); which ensure that body signs of distress are systematically overriden (*step 2*) and that the body uses the organ in a harmful or non-synchronized way and which prevent the body's immune system from providing adequate protection in that organ (*step 3*). Further, we know that the more chronic and routine these habits are, the more at risk the individual is.

We have also identified the psychological patterns attached to these habits and looked at the kind of body-mind networks that constitute the 'worst-case' risk. We know that someone at high risk usually has bad habits focused on a single organ (or organ system) and that this becomes a symbol for the expression of most of their emotional activity. We know that the person who actually develops cancer usually does so when the three stages of risk occur together as a systematic part of his or her personality and lifestyle. Lastly, we know that the relationships an individual has play a far more significant role than in other illnesses in determining whether or not an individual falls into the three-level risk pattern. In short, we can pinpoint habits of *behaviour* that result in carcinogen exposure, habits of *internal avoidance* that result in override and habitual *psychological* states that result in a helpless, depressed and fatigue-ridden reaction to stress (and lowered immunity).

Now, we are all exposed to these risks from time to time. Let's therefore identify those kinds of people who should think about prevention:

• The individual who is at risk at any *one* of the risk stages (the low cancer risk)
• The individual at risk at *two* levels (the moderate cancer risk)
• The individual at risk at all *three* levels (the high risk person).

We'll examine each in turn, identify the kinds of habits creating the risk, warn about what can happen if these habits aren't attended to, look at the problems in personality that might be causing them, and suggest ways and means of tackling them.

People at low cancer risk   First, if you routinely engage in any activity that exposes you to a carcinogen you are at risk and you'll have to sit up and take notice. If you work in a high-risk industry, if you're a miner, a furniture worker, exposed to asbestos, if you're a bar-tender or sell alcohol, if you're a smoker, if you have ulcerative colitis or Crohn's disease, a gastric ulcer, cystitis or fibroaedomas, or are prone to benign breast tumours, or if you have a chronic cough or chronically over-indulge in sun-bathing — if any of these conditions apply to you then you are probably at risk. But it's a low risk, similar to the risk you take if you drive when tired; you'll survive as long as nothing unexpected goes wrong.

Similarly, if you routinely subject your body to abnormal levels of override where you ignore its signs of discomfort and stress, you are exposing yourself to a low risk. Even if you don't smoke, don't work with asbestos or have indigestion, the fact of *routinely* exhausting any of your body's organs, lowering their ability to function, or if you operate an organ or organ system out of synch with other body systems, all can put you at risk. So, for example, if you're chronically constipated, have chronic indigestion or stomach ache, but continue to try to function as normal, you're at risk. If you are chronically unfit or under-exercised and yet you try to behave as if you were fit by driving your body to limits it can't cope with, you will be vulnerable; ditto if you are chronically under-exercised and you avoid situations where you should be *healthily* stressed or fatigued.

Lastly, if you are prone to insecurity, feel isolated most of the time, feel chronically fatigued and without stamina, take care; you are likely to lower your ability to cope with life's problems. You might be fine and live to an old age, but then again, too much will depend on the stability of your circumstances and too little on your body's innate ability to protect itself.

Remember, any one of these conditions leaves your marginally vulnerable. To achieve the healthy body-mind relationship that I described in the last chapter, you have to *use* your body and *use* it properly most of the time. Bad habits are permissible provided (a) they don't become chronic, (b) they aren't the *only* thing you use to express distress or emotions. As we saw earlier, bad habits like smoking, bad overrides like constipation, avoiding key areas of living like intimacy, even episodes of isolation, loneliness, depression, fatigue, and so on, can on occasion be useful and necessary *if* they are being used as a catalyst to achieve something else. For example, after the death of someone close, or when a deep relationship goes sour, one is liable to feel miserable; the body's resistance and immunity will be lowered. Such a person will be at risk, especially if he or she also smokes or drinks as part of being grief-stricken. But so long as grieving is properly felt, that is, if one *also* cries, re-thinks, feels upset, *feels* lonely, and so on, your body will cope. Note that there's a difference between *feeling* lonely and *being* lonely; many people aren't alone in the physical sense, but they can be lonely and deny it. Provided the grief is 'going somewhere' and does not become either chronic or passive, i.e. with no emotional experiences, grief can be an incredibly valuable experience. In fact, if under the correct circumstances you cannot grieve properly, if you don't *collapse* properly, you could be in a lot of physiological and psychological trouble.

To take a second example, if you have to face an episode of unusual tension such as taking an exam, you might smoke excessively to calm your nerves; you might work far too hard, stay awake too late, take no exercise or eat junk food, but so long as this happens only for some specific, useful cause, soon ends and you return to healthy normality quickly, you'll survive. In fact, many of us need these episodes to live properly.

The danger signs to watch out for

- Behaviours that become too routine: if there is no reversion to normal after a crisis or a catalytic episode, and certain behaviours insidiously become a permanent part of your life. *Chronic* means something persistently used day after day, week after week. It means that you can't stop it any time you want — if you try, you fail. If you are unable to stop any habit for a period of two months then you're at risk.

- When your habits become your only emotional outlets — then you are at risk. Thus, for example, if you have a bad cold which is making you feel miserable and all you do about it is smoke more and more — that's dangerous; you're expressing your irritation and crossness with the cold by harming yourself further. If, when you get upset, all you do is reach for a cigarette, you're at risk. By the same token, if the only time you ever show anger is by being impatient with your bowel action when constipated, and you tear yourself or otherwise hurt yourself, it can be dangerous. If all you ever do to show your emotions is misuse your body or let it be misused, as for example, in love-making, you're in the same boat.

- If you are a very unemotional person, you could be at risk. If you *feel* angry, hostile, upset, tense, loving, warm, needy, but never *show* these feelings, then you should take note. It's worse if you vaguely feel all or some of these things but never actually *talk* about them, or acknowledge them to yourself.
- If you chronically lack stamina, you're at risk. No one should routinely feel that everything is too much effort. You shouldn't *always* be tired. It is worse if you can never manage to exert yourself and worse still if you always have an excuse for never doing anything.

What can happen if you are at risk from such behaviours? Three basic things. First, you could be vulnerable to growing psychological habituation, i.e. become dependent on the habit. Once a habit or an emotion-denying pattern is established as a part of your daily life, it becomes harder and harder to shift it on your own. As it is always present, it becomes impossible to tell how much a part of your life it is, or how much you actually engage in it. Inevitably you slip into relying on it more and more, and you can then also become vulnerable to the second and third factors that follow.

Second, you can become too dependent on those around you for your survival. In other words, you may rely on others to *control* your habits — someone important to you (husband, wife, mother, father), to nag about keeping your weight down or controlling your smoking. Should you suddenly lose that person and be unable to replace that person's monitoring of your behaviour, then you might suddenly have problems. It may become far worse if the checks or balances provided by your partner are part of a subtextual game you play, whereby you defy him or her and then alternately resist or submit, depending on what is going on underneath; the habit, then, can easily replace proper intimacy and the proper expression of emotion. I'm thinking here of the case where a couple act out their problems or differences in personality by concentrating on bad habits like smoking; one partner might, for example, resist the good intentions of the other ('that's enough for today') either openly or in secret because he or she feels that the other's intentions are really motivated out of dislike, irritation or frustration.

Lastly, you can become over-dependent on pure chance to an extent where an outside stroke of luck, say, a bad illness, an accident, or loss of a job, will expose your lack of physical stamina and preparedness. If, at the same time, you were to lose any moderating relationship, you would be doubly at risk. For some people, such events 'shake them up' in the right way and they are able to change for the better. If you cannot change your patterns, then you're in trouble. How often have you heard people say, 'Oh, everything was fine. I was on top of the world until the car crash, then I lost my job, my husband/wife walked out on me and I fell ill'? Everything *was* all right, but it was only all right because the supporting external circumstances were favourable. The real test of a healthy individual is not if he or she can sail through life with everything being 'all right', but whether or not their body-mind systems can cope when external supports collapse or they have a run of bad luck. When real-life problems strike far too many people find their day-to-day habits are simply not up to the stress involved, at which point, any long-standing vulnerability emerges.

What to do? If you don't want to spend time looking at yourself in depth, then just trying to give up a bad habit might help. At best you might discover the discipline or will-power to do so. At worst, you'll join the multitude who give up bad habits for set periods of time, then relapse, then try a new cure, and so on *ad infinitum*; all of which at least help to break the routine.

The best form of prevention however is to take the time to look at yourself thoroughly and try to see why and how you do things. Try to understand what goes on in your body and in your mind. See if there aren't, in fact, signs already present that you could act on; try broadening out, try other ways of coping with your problems. Talk to people; talking about your problems is the first step towards self-recognition and self-knowledge. Take advice and ideas from others and try them out. Above all, try breaking your risk patterning with episodes, perhaps, of not smoking. Try to identify situations that cause you to feel tense and then try new ways of coping with both the situation and your tension.

What you actually do about this depends, of course, on your individual circumstances and it would be wrong of me to try to guide you in any specific direction. What I can do though, is ask you to remember the points above. If you do have risky habits, you are exposing your body to danger and you shouldn't leave it in this state. If you make a concerted effort and do something substantial using whatever methods you choose, you will help remove the risk. At this level of risk, there really is a simple cause-effect relationship between your habits and most individuals can see this and help themselves. If you can't, seek some other form of help. You might also read on and look at some of the tactics I suggest for people in the other risk categories.

People at moderate cancer risk   If you've read the preceding section and you feel that pretty much *all* the material presented there is true of you, then you are probably a moderate risk already; if you have a fixation about a specific habit, and routinely override your body signs of discomfort, that puts you in the moderate risk bracket. Low risk occurs when you are guilty of one or two of the bad habits mentioned. To qualify as 'moderate' look out for the following in addition to the signs already mentioned for the low-risk category.

The danger signs

- Are you unable to think about getting through the day without your special habits? Like Burt in Chapter 4, if the first thing you do in the morning is reach for a cigarette or, like Carole, take a laxative, then your habit has become too much a part of your life.
- Are you never without some form of discomfort? When was the last time you woke up without pain, tension, or a 'lost' feeling, as if you've lost track of your body? These are all symptoms of a lowered level of resistance, and lowered attention to the body. We all have aches and pains, but nine times out of ten they are for highly specific and temporary reasons; a headache or backache, for example, may be due to holding certain muscle groups in tension for too long, insom-

nia may be through worrying about an upcoming event, muscle ache or pain may arise after bruising exercise, a stomach ache may be the result of failing to go to the toilet when you should have. We can trace the discomforts back to their source and usually do something about them. It is when such discomforts are present every day, wearing you down, that they constitute a danger sign.

- Are you beginning to hate your body, or parts of it? I don't mean in the sense of not liking your ears or the size of your nose, but actually feeling disgust or shame at a part of yourself: breasts, stomach, chest, sex organs, or whatever. The mere act of disliking a particular part of you won't, obviously, cause cancer, but it's a useful warning signal. If this is the case, you should be careful that you aren't allowing bad and risky habits to form, involving neglect of the part you don't like, misuse of the organ, or anything that will create a vulnerability in that area.
- Do you feel lethargic more times than not? If you can't remember when you didn't feel tired, have no stamina and no energy day in and day out, you are at risk.
- Do you feel that the tension inside you is unbearable any longer? And worse, do you feel there is nothing to be done about it?

If you can answer yes to most of these questions, it is more than likely that you already have, or are very close to developing, cancer. It would be very wise to have medical check-ups regularly and to get help early if necessary. There are, of course, exceptions. Some people exhibit all the symptoms and habits I've described without having cancer and, of course, there are those who exhibit all these symptoms but have some other illness — most often a heart condition. By and large, it is more likely that the chronic exposure to carcinogens, the chronic over-focusing on a specific organ, and the avoidance of proper body-mind emotional activity will have resulted in changes to cell structure in the organ. Whether or not these changes have created an identifiable tumour will probably depend on how chronic the habits are and the quality of your immune functioning.

What to do?   First, keep an eye on your vital signs; look out for the changes we traditionally associate with the presence of an identifiable tumour. The American Medical Association lists the following seven early warning signs:

- A thickening or lump in any area, particularly the breast
- A change in bowel or bladder habits
- An irritating cough or persistent hoarseness
- An ulcer or a sore that does not heal
- Unusual discharge or unusual bleeding
- A change in a wart or a mole
- Difficulty in swallowing, or indigestion

If you find anything, see your doctor for help and advice. If you are a moderate or high-risk personality, prompt action at this point can achieve a great deal. Many cancers, if spotted early, respond very well to treatment.

The second step you must take is to start work on modifying your habits. Whatever organ system is affected must be attended to. If you smoke, for example, now is the time to cut down or modify your pattern; if you have stomach, digestive, bowel or urinary problems, now is the time to change your eating habits; if you have many lovers and a chronic vaginal or penile discharge, now is the time to do something about your patterns of intimacy and how you see yourself.

People in this category must recognize that they need help. Your doctor is the first person to seek out, and again the act of talking things over can help; reading up about the effects of diet, alcohol and tobacco on your health may take you a step further in doing something about your habits. Seeing a dietician, or someone with experience of carcinogens, can be invaluable; taking a course in relaxation, meditation, hypnosis, or similar techniques can help 'loosen you up' and lower levels of tension; talking to a psychologist, behaviour therapist, or psychiatrist can help you achieve better insights into yourself and teach you ways of coping with old habits. The point is, take responsibility for yourself; do or see whatever or whoever you want, as long as the result is effective.

On a note of caution, there is always the possibility that

some of the help offered will be of no use to you. I, and I'm sure many of my colleagues, have had the experience of sending a patient for medical help and later finding that the medication prescribed by a GP had been misused by the patient to the extent that he or she had become dependent on it. It was nobody's 'fault' as such; each 'helper' thought he or she was doing the correct thing, and the patient thought it was all right to become dependent.

When it comes to *preventive* medicine for cancer you are the best person to do the job, if you know where to look. Remember, most medical units are trained to cope with problems which already exist and your GP is keyed to helping you with specific ailments. In current medical practice, preventive action for cancer is minimal; few doctors have enough time to devote to patients with established medical problems, let alone to think about what 'might be'. In fact, I believe this to be part of the reason why cancer and heart conditions have become such big killers; reducing the number of victims involves a great deal of preventive work, much of which lies outside the scope of current medical practice. I'm convinced too that the burgeoning interest in alternative medicine is partly due to the fact that conventional medicine is not yet properly geared to cope with the kind of preventive re-training required by people prone to cancer or heart-attacks. Many people want help with a myriad of minor ailments: constipation, body ache, back ache, tension, and so on — all of them within the scope of alternative medicine. They know their GPs are busy, that hospitals are engaged in *vital* activities, like heart surgery, liver transplants and casualties, so they look for simple, 'folk' cures and a sympathetic ear. Often they are able to find both.

I believe it should be our responsibility as practitioners and patients to help each other far more than we do at present, or have done in the past. Cancer prevention is a very real possibility — hence this book and others like it. Bear in mind that helping yourself is a major part of the prevention task, in marked contrast to the almost minor role you will play if you land up in hospital being treated for cancer; if you value your own freedom of action, act now while you still can.

People at high cancer risk   All the warning signs described for the low and moderate risk conditions apply to people who are at high risk. I am sure you will appreciate that the difference between the three risk stages is very much a matter of degree. If you're not sure where you fall, focus on the general high-risk pattern, and if you feel that it does, in large part, define you, then consider yourself a high risk. Of course, whatever your risk level, it is not healthy to leave *chronic* bad habits unattended. If you're looking for one single determining factor of high or low risk then *chronicity* is the thing to look out for. With that established we can take a look at the model I have found most useful for self-helping and reducing cancer risk.

A preventive strategy: Six steps to cancer prevention   If we're going to change this high-risk picture, six key things need to be done.

1 The carcinogen-exposing habits have to be modified, if not eliminated altogether.
2 You have to learn new ways of attending to your body 'sounds'. As a first step, if you can't 'hear' them because you've ignored them for so long, just starting to listen will help.
3 You must learn to devote more time to yourself.
4 You have to improve the operating level of whichever organ you have tended to focus on.
5 You must learn to relate to people better, to see yourself more realistically, and learn to use your body-mind systems more robustly.
6 You have to learn to cope with normal stress and upset more healthily.

All this amounts to a complete overhaul of your personality and your body. However, I'm well aware that not everyone can achieve that so with each step I'll explain what to do and hope that you'll travel as far as possible along the route. At the very least, achieving the first three steps will help you reduce your risk from high to moderate. It's up to you.

The *basic strategy* involved here is quite simple; over a

period of time you've coped with problems in your life by locking your body-mind systems into an unhealthy pattern in which your body state is reinforced by tight emotional control, and by your psychological blandness and helplessness. Your mind, as it were, has been put into suspended animation and can't free itself from this body-mind pattern. You must begin by making both psychological and behavioural changes.

If you were to make changes in your habits in line with preventive step 1, (perhaps try to stop smoking), what would happen? Answer — you'd experience increased awareness of your internal body state: you'd feel panicked, afraid, maybe a little hopeful. You'd concentrate on getting through the day and start worrying about what you're going to do without the habit. All these events are just the material you'd need to work on preventive step 2 — learning to use your intelligence *to listen* to your internal state.

Preventive step 3 would force you to attend to your organs and your internal state more carefully and encourage you to develop better ways of dealing with them; you'd have to concentrate on how you felt inside and act on what you found. This in turn would throw up emotional and physiological issues that you would have to tackle in preventive steps 5 and 6. Each step creates the momentum for the next, until ultimately you would arrive at the point where you would have to improve your interpersonal activity in order to cope with the emotions and feelings released in preventive steps 5 and 6.

To recap, we start by changing your habits and finish by altering your psychological awareness. We disrupt your bad habits and the resulting body-mind turmoil is our raw material; we want to break it up into its elements and then put it all back together again in a much healthier way.

Let me give you a brief example as an illustration, and then go on to look at a fuller case study to see how it can work in practice.

Let's assume we're dealing with an individual who meets all our high-risk conditions and let's say the problem area is in the bowel region and shows up as chronic constipation. Preventive steps 1 and 2 would involve focusing on the constipation and linking it to stressful events. We would teach the individual to

(a) recognize the stressful situations that block the normal sphincter relaxation response, and (b) to recognize the alternative and competing body feelings that automatically precede the act (discomfort, full bowel, etc.). Preventive *step 3* would involve learning how to create ideal conditions, such as quietness and privacy, re-learning how to relax properly, and building these into daily life. These three steps would undoubtedly throw up anxieties, resentment, even hostility about doing this, which in preventive *step 4* would have to be attended to so that the individual would listen more to the natural early signs of bowel tension or discomfort and act on them, rather than to the pressure of time or worry. Once a person recognizes the conflict inside, he or she has to be taught to *attend* to it and to disregard other psychological pressures; getting private time allows this. In preventive *steps 5 and 6* the individual would have to learn to deal with these conflicts separately and build up the necessary relationships required to permit the changes to become permanent, so that being upset resulted, not in a frozen bowel action, but in showing emotion or upset in some other way and to another person. In other words, this remedial action would free the central nervous sympathetic system monitoring bowel action from being distracted by irrelevancies.

The best way to illustrate how this six-step strategy works in practice is to describe how it applies in a specific person; so let's look at Allan, a forty-year-old engineer with a smoking problem, and many of Burt's characteristics.

Allan was clearly a high-risk person. He'd been smoking for years, with a recurrent bronchial infection caused by this and his low general immunity. It settled in every winter and took several months to improve, and while he was always on the verge of giving up smoking, he never did. As a partial insomniac, he smoked eighteen to twenty hours a day. In a sense his smoking habits formed the core of his existence. Married with three children, he worked very hard, was relatively successful and seemed a very calm, reassuring person. Only by studying his smoking behaviour could you really detect the inner tensions that were there. Originally he came to see me to help him stop smoking, but we were able to achieve rather more than that.

Preventive step 1: Breaking up habits   After getting to know
Allan and his background, we set about identifying the kind of
breathing habits that I felt were a source of risk. Where he was
going wrong in his use of smoking was that he was having (a) no
breaks from it (b) he was using it at times when his body state
clearly demanded he shouldn't — when he had a cough, when he
was racing upstairs to a meeting, and so on. Moreover I felt his
smoking had formed a barrier between himself and his wife; she
felt that he 'smelt' of smoke, so it put her off him and this often
interfered with their closeness, particularly their sexual
intimacy. She said that he nearly always wanted to smoke as
soon as he had ejaculated; she felt pressured to orgasm quickly
because of this, which in turn discouraged her from other forms
of physical contact.

I saw no point in trying to get Allan to give up the habit
immediately because firstly, he had nothing to replace it with,
secondly he didn't know why he smoked ('automatic,' he said,
'I've always done it'), and thirdly he said he was quite unaware
of what he did with his cigarette smoking, i.e. expressing
nervousness, anger, fear, and so on. If he'd concentrated on
stopping, I felt sure he'd start again as soon as he was no longer
seeing me and was free of the pressure to stop. So we did some
habit-breaking experiments to explore his habit in detail.

First, I sat him down in a chair in my office and asked him
not to smoke for one minute. For a while he sat there smiling,
relaxed and a bit puzzled, but then he began to show body signs
of intense discomfort: he fidgeted in his chair, said his hands felt
clammy, kept looking at his watch, and so on. The first time we
tried it, he denied that he'd felt 'uncomfortable' (his bland
inattention to his body was at work), but as we kept on with the
experiment he began to admit that he felt an enormous weight
on him: 'It seems such a long period of time, that minute. I don't
know what to do with myself. I don't know what to do with the
silence. I feel I ought to be doing something else.' Another thing I
noticed was the way he waited for my approval before admitting
what he was feeling; he had 'expected' me to think and see
things as he did and was very relieved to find that it was okay to
say he felt tense, that, in fact, it was a normal reaction.

Then I suggested that he stop smoking at *selected times*, in particular, whenever he was doing something physically demanding (*overriding* his body's demand for extra, clean air), thus ensuring that the worst effects of body stress were reduced. I also suggested that he stop for a set period after having intercourse with his wife — thus ensuring that he focus on her needs and wants more. Lastly, I suggested that he practice stopping smoking for just one minute in every hour so that he could get used to the uncomfortable feelings that arose inside himself.

This simple-sounding programme achieved quite a lot. Initially Allan was somewhat antagonistic (I felt) about the whole idea of asking for help and stopping smoking. On the surface he said he wanted to stop smoking, but he approached it from a more defiant stance inside — as if saying 'I dare you to stop me'. When I reassured him that we would come at it differently, that it was more important to change *how* he smoked rather than simply to *stop* smoking, he felt more co-operative.

What did we achieve in preventive step one? Well, for a start, Allan found that not smoking while doing something energetic was a great relief. 'I can work on something without getting my eyes full of smoke. It seems so silly, so logical, but I wouldn't have thought to do it on my own. Running upstairs or to catch a train isn't such an effort if you're not smoking.' It was a small but significant gain because he was quickly able to establish this as a routine.

When it came to intimacy, he admitted that he felt quite ashamed of what he'd been doing to his wife (putting pressure on her to 'get it over with quickly'), and that after a few times, he had found his wife more responsive and more physically affectionate afterwards, which he liked. He himself took this a step further by ensuring he took a shower before they made love so, in his words, 'I smell sweeter'. By not focusing on smoking he found he had more *conscious* time to think about love-making, his wife and so on, and that he could participate more in the enjoyment of having made love. 'Previously,' he said, 'sure I wanted to make love, but then, once I'd come, straight away, I'd want to smoke and I'd forget about my wife.' Now he actually began to take more part in their intimacy; he began to enjoy post-coital feelings and remarked that they are a very important part of having sex. Once established, he said he didn't know why he'd smoked in the past — 'the feeling of enjoyment and love is so potent I wouldn't want to spoil it by thinking about smoking.'

For the purposes of our programme though, by far the biggest impact was in the non-smoking minute I'd asked him to practise. This took us on to preventive step two:

Preventive step 2: Attending to body sounds   What I was trying to get Allan to do in this experiment was to start 'listening' to his body 'sounds'. First, he had to face up to the tensions and pressures inside him that he concealed by the act of smoking. Second, he had to face the source of those tensions outside himself, i.e. in the world, or the context in which he lived. Third, he had to start 'listening' and attending to the discomfort his body was experiencing (his override) while he was smoking.

We very quickly established the first and third aims; Allan, in fact, became quite voluble about what was going on inside himself; 'Right. I'm waiting for a meeting to start. I reach for a cigarette then I remember I must wait for one minute. My foot starts tapping, I'm impatient, I want the cigarette. I begin to wonder why my foot is tapping — why I feel so panicked. I notice my breathing is heavy. My throat is sore and I'm wheezing a bit. I try to take a deep breath to calm myself (which is what I'd do if I was smoking). The air's nice but it's painful. The minute's up. Thank God.'

Linking these experiences, especially the tension, to something like the meeting, was a lot more difficult. He'd think about the question, look puzzled and then say: 'There's no one there to worry about. It was just a routine meeting; I wasn't nervous.' But soon he began to make the links. It wasn't the people in the meeting (he was friendly with them all), but the act of talking to so many people at once. He felt awkward, self-conscious and worse, silly, just admitting this to me. But it was true and by studying his non-smoking minute records in a variety of situations it was clear that he felt a low-level sense of insecurity and inadequacy almost constantly. He became very worried when he realized the extent of his insecurity and had a very bad week thinking that it meant he was 'insane', but I reassured him that it was normal to feel insecure, and *abnormal* to hide those feelings from himself and everyone else; it isolated him, distanced him from people. By not sharing or admitting to his anxieties, he had no way of thinking about them, no framework for discussion, for trying to learn from others different possible ways of coping.

This is a very important point. Allan came from a family which censured the discussion and expression of emotion and he found that this had imposed a block on his development in this area. As he knew no other way of 'being', he didn't even realize his deficiency. In other areas — in conversation, in thinking, in general behaviour — he had developed as a normal person would without being aware that emotionally-normal people actually feel, talk about, experiment with emotions just as he might talk about the weather or a maths problem. I nearly always found cancer people stuck at what one could call a child's level of thinking about emotions, but once released from their restrictions and aware of their right to express and play with emotions just like anyone else, they progressed rapidly to a more open, self-exploratory state. Allan considered it 'unmanly' or 'silly' to show upset or fear, and he couldn't really see at first that this was a result of never being allowed to be afraid or 'unmanly' and so find out what it all meant. We went on to preventive step 3 to explore this.

Preventive step 3: giving yourself more time   Allan had never been given time at home to discuss how he felt about things. Consequently he didn't give himself time to think about his 'weaknesses', as he called emotions, and he didn't give other people, like his wife, time either. By the same token he wasn't given much time to be sick, to be affectionate, and so on, so he didn't give himself much time to listen to his own sicknesses or to his own needs for affection. His view of reality was very much defined by rational tasks: he had a company to run, jobs to do at home, the task of looking after his family, all of which he did well. But there was one missing factor: he had never been taught to tackle the *task* of looking after himself.

With his growing awareness of his body discomfort and his realization of the constant tension he felt inside, Allan needed time to make sense out of them, to organize and probe his feelings. One way I used of showing him how to do this was to ask him to find half an hour each weekend in which to do nothing but sit quietly and think about himself locked in his room. The first time he just couldn't do it: 'There was so much to do around the house, honestly, I felt so guilty just being so self-centred.'

The second time he managed to do it but he couldn't focus on himself; he found a hundred other things to think about. The third time though, it worked; 'I suddenly realized how tired I was. I'd been smoking, my lungs ached, I'd just finished a report and I was due to go to my parents for supper and suddenly it was all too much. I felt like my head was exploding. I nearly cried.'

Actually Allan was feeling sorry for himself and it was very important to encourage him to do so because often, just behind the bland facade, lies a great wall of self-pity and underneath that, a lot of undirected anger. 'Slowly I began to realize how depressed I felt about myself; I work hard, have a lung problem, I never take a holiday, never have fun, I'm overweight. But if I think about it too long I get so steamed up inside I think I'll hit someone.'

What this did for Allan was to make him 'listen' to himself; it gave him his own 'personal' time and taught him to keep on wanting that time too. It was simple conditioning and he soon got used to the idea, eventually spending at least half an hour a day on himself.

Preventive step 4: Improving the target organ's functioning
By now Allan was well on the way to a cure. At the *somatic* level he was beginning to feel physically better; the reduction in smoking improved his bronchial infection, his closer contact with his wife and his better general breathing helped him to feel what it would be like to have a healthy breathing apparatus.

At the *psychological* level he was feeling very disturbed about himself and his emotions. He still clung to his smoking behaviour, but he was shaken. He was also beginning to sense the links between his nervous state and his smoking habit.

Now, having established all these new awarenesses, we wanted to improve how he used his breathing. I suggested that he could now well afford to do some exercise every day. I linked this to his daily half hour of 'private time' and explored it as a first step in actually looking after his body better and of learning to attend to his body symptoms. His lungs were painful? 'Fine,' I said, 'then let's do something about that by doing breathing exercises to help you clear them. Let's do some exercise to improve their efficiency and in the process let's help you to keep fit by dieting and so lose weight.' Put like that, how could he refuse? And so his half hour became an hour a day devoted to himself. His breathing slowly improved, his weight dropped, he felt better and he felt proud because he'd done it by himself. Once he'd established this new behaviour as a routine part of his life, I encouraged him to play a sport to further improve his breathing and the co-ordination of his lungs with the rest of his body. After this, his bronchial infection really improved. While he found all these new developments quite anxiety-provoking (he worried lest he be neglecting his family or his job) the gains in his lung-efficiency were so significant that he accepted it. Also, while exercising, while thinking about himself, while playing sport, there wasn't time to smoke. Thus gradually the number of hours a day he wasn't smoking had greatly increased.

Preventive step 5: Improving interpersonal relationships   At this stage Allan still hadn't changed how he coped with emotions, or how he coped with stress. He still did not talk openly to his wife, and he still had a bland exterior. Now it became a question of actually doing something about the level at which he made contact with people. The first thing I suggested he do was to start talking to his wife about what he thought and felt in the hour he spent alone. He found this very difficult and so I saw them together a few times to help him overcome his nervousness.

What emerged was how much she felt the need to talk; she was longing to open up, but was shy and a little timid in the face of his personality. Not only had he blocked off his own experience of emotions, but had unintentionally inhibited her expression. Given the opportunity to talk about feelings, she just poured out a mass of ideas and insights she had never been able to discuss with anyone. I think while Allan was overwhelmed, he was also delighted and after two sessions of mutual discovery, I left them to it.

However, these achievements were largely verbal. How did Allan manage the fact that as an adult in mid-life he didn't know the first thing about feeling angry. How did he suddenly learn to express emotions when he felt upset after forty years of learning to do the opposite?

The answer was and is that one has to use trial and error with someone very close until one gets it right. No one is too old to learn and Allan started with me, then with his wife. Let me tell you about one episode.

He had to wait to see me for an appointment. When he came in he was smoking and he instantly started blowing smoke everywhere. I knew he was angry. So I said: 'You're angry.'

'No I'm not,' he said, angrily.

'I'm sure you are, Allan, so why don't you put your cigarette out and shout at me?' He wouldn't, but I persisted and sure enough he was angry, but he didn't know how to shout. Nor could he look at me while he shouted; it contradicted his bland assurance that he wasn't angry. So we practised until he learned to shout and this helped him a lot. He felt relieved that I didn't mind if he shouted; he enjoyed shouting and being angry even if he felt an idiot while doing it.

I could help him with his anger but I could do nothing about teaching him how to cry, be comforted and so on. I needn't have worried, his wife did that. One day she just knew that he was upset so she bullied him into *being* upset until he succumbed.

You would not believe the number of people in this world who don't know how to be angry, to shout, to cry or to laugh, and need to be helped to learn how to do so. Much of my work involves teaching people the basics of emotional existence. Not only does this help them achieve a better relationship with their partners, but it is absolutely vital for their body functioning. In Allan's case, allowing himself to recognize and talk about being upset and to learn to actually *be* upset meant that a new body-mind pattern had begun to take shape. Previously Allan's cycle of body-mind functioning went something like this:

Internal need	*Internal body-mind state*	*Habit*
Anxiety ⎫		
Tension ⎬ →	High arousal →	Smoking
Fear ⎭	High stress	

His new cycle went like this:

Internal need	*Internal body-mind state*	*Habit*
Anxiety ⎫		Becoming upset
Tension ⎬ →	High arousal →	Talking it over
Fear ⎭	High stress	Being comforted

You can see that the early cycle did absolutely nothing for his internal body-mind state while the newer one did; smoking gives a minor 'high' and minor comfort quite unrelated to the degree of stress and arousal existing in the body. Allan's new habits were a far more thorough-going and natural means of attending to his internal state. This is what babies and animals do and what we adults should all learn to do quite regularly. Crying or sharing your upset is physically much better for you, builds a healthier body, healthier relationships and a healthier mind than smoking ever will.

Expressing emotions will not automatically solve all your problems. Expressing emotions very often creates problems in the sense that, once expressed, you and those around you have to cope with what emerges. Very often, when you begin to express yourself, you do so very crudely; you get too cross, too upset and you will not really be at all satisfied intellectually. You need practice and often a guiding hand, which is one reason why a psychologist might be able to help at this point. By the same token, I'm also not suggesting that you walk around 'letting it all hang out' as the hippies used to say; the effective expression of emotion demands that you learn how to express the right emotion in the right context. Like learning to get a golf shot right, it takes a knowledge of when to be soft, when to hit hard and so on. You also have to learn with whom you can and cannot be emotional: it's no good weeping all over your boss! All this takes time and patience and practice. While you're getting practice, remember that you're releasing the air in the pressure cooker inside you. You might not like what comes out, but it is the meat and drink of proper living and, of course, of proper intimate relationships. Partners in life should base much of their private activity together on exploring the recesses of their minds and emotions; it's what loving is all about.

Allan and his wife really worked hard at breaking up his habits and deepening their intimacy; once I'd explained to them both how vital it was to make their emotional life work, they got stuck in. By building up their contact, I knew the pressure on Allan (that is, his internal state) would subside; he would feel routinely less tense. This, plus the sheer pleasure he discovered in his new breathing habits, served to reduce his smoking. He didn't stop, but he cut down enormously and above all, he restricted his smoking to occasions when he really felt like it. More importantly, he began to take more responsibility for himself and his health.

Preventive step 6: coping with normal stress   Of course all Allan's new behaviours worked well until he hit one of life's bumps; his company ran into trouble and a real crisis began for him. Promptly he reverted to his old bland self and his pattern of chain-smoking. Fortunately for him, his wife rebelled. She threatened to leave him if he didn't get back to the new 'person' he'd become. Faced with threats from his wife and the crisis at work he came to me again for help. My advice to him was: 'It's no good hoping crises in life won't crop up. They always do. But if you have built up an open supportive relationship with your partner it will sustain you in a crisis. If you have built up a proper co-operation in your body-mind system, if you are fit and healthy, your body will support you. If you have kept up your new habits of emotional expression, they will support you. Try to trust all your new learning; smoke if you must, but don't stop anything else. Keep exercising, keep talking to yourself, keep to your private time, keep showing your feelings to your wife, cry. If that is how upset you feel, it will strengthen your ability to cope.'

This, I think, is the nub of the whole programme; when normal stressful situations crop up, you *need* a healthy intimacy, a healthy body-mind framework, and a healthy set of coping habits. The *worst* time to give them up is under the pressure of normal crises. Remember, learning new behaviours is not going to stop you having problems. However, it will change how you solve your problems and how they affect you.

Allan wasn't easily convinced and it was a few months before he stabilized. He was soon back to his high point and much wiser. I feel sure that a crisis won't affect Allan so traumatically again. Perhaps his crisis came too soon after his new learning?

Well, that's the six-step preventive model. I couldn't guarantee to Allan that he would never develop cancer, but we could be pretty sure that he was seriously trying to take every possible step to lower his risk significantly. Whatever happens in the future, he is considerably better placed to cope than he used to be.

It also needs to be said that if people were made more aware of cancer risks in general and the preventive tasks that can be carried out much earlier on in life, far fewer people would suffer from cancer. Let me give you some indication of the kind of preventive programme that would, I think, greatly help in alerting people to the kinds of risks they face and how they can be minimized.

SOCIETY AND CANCER PREVENTION

Society already does a fair amount to alert the public to cancer risks; the campaign against smoking conducted by certain civic groups and the medical professions in some countries is perhaps the most public form this has taken, but there are others. Action by food and drug-scrutinizing agencies in the US and UK has resulted in lowered risks from exposure to carcinogens in what we eat and drink; campaigns against the risks of radiation from nuclear plants and other forms of irradiation have similarly helped to draw attention to both the risks attached to exposure and the need for greater protection for workers than was previously the case. Similarly, environmentalist groups concerned with lowering air, soil and water pollution help to alert the public to cancer risks from these sources.

As a general measure, this focusing on carcinogens and trying to reduce the public's exposure to them is a vitally necessary part of cancer prevention. Current reseach into the subtler effects of, say, cigarette smoke and exhaust fumes on people, will help to increase public knowledge and awareness of the air we breathe.

Improved cancer screening techniques, like the Pap smear for cervical cancer, approach the problem differently, but are just as effective in lowering cancer risks. Their aim is to detect cancer or pre-cancerous changes in body tissue early, so that treatment can be given more promptly with a corresponding improvement in its effectiveness. Another thing that is changing the public's risk from cancer is the interest in health and physical fitness; coupled with better thinking about diets and eating habits, these go a long way towards improving the ability of the individual to fight cancer and, of course, many other diseases.

However, I think we can go further. If you look at the model presented in this book, you see that exposure to carcinogens is only one of three factors that need to be present for cancer to form. The habits associated with overriding discomfort and lowering immunity play as vital a role, and in high-risk people, their psychological and emotional states enter into the picture as well; high-risk people tend to perform all the wrong risk-habits all at the same time.

If we could alert the public to the presence of these other factors as much as they have been alerted to the dangers of carcinogens, I think a far more safety-conscious attitude to cancer would result. I know from my own clinical experience with people like Allan that much of the propaganda against tobacco smoke has no effect on many smokers' actual behaviour. Encouraging people to think about modifying *how* they smoke and to think about modifying how they care for their lungs in general (and not just focusing on giving up smoking) is another way of encouraging them to change.

We also need to make people more aware of the role played in cancer development by what may seem minor, and irritating, bad habits. We may be so used to chronic constipation, indigestion, bladder, bowel and genital tract infections, chronic lethargy, chronic avoidance of emotions and poor interpersonal contact that we hardly consider them important. Yet they can be crucial if they occur in the contexts described in this book. Exposure to carcinogens plus exposure to some of these habits is a little like writing a prescription for the development of cancer.

At the practical level, two additional notions ought to be propagated to the public about cancer. The first would encourage much greater awareness of *other* bad habits (described above) that can predispose an individual to cancer. We need to inform people about what can go wrong if they persist with chronic lethargy, constipation or stress. People need to know that there are things that can be done to remedy such ailments. Help available from professionals includes behaviour therapy, psychotherapy and counselling at the most practical of levels. Again, the earlier one starts, the better the results. As a society, I feel we should use the psychologist or psychiatrist in the same way as a GP — someone you go to for minor practical ailments. The overwhelming stigma attached to seeing 'a shrink' has had most unfortunate consequences; psychologists' and psychiatrists' jobs would be a lot easier if 'normal' people consulted them long before their 'normal problems' became obsessions, The benefits of psychology and psychiatry should not be reserved for the mentally ill alone; quite apart from the fact that there may be more disturbed people outside mental homes than in them, coping with modern living demands practical advice from time to time. Just as you'd consult an expert technician to fix your computer or car so you should be able to see a psychologist to help you over a hurdle or two.

There is another side to this. Certainly, one should feel freer to seek psychological help, but if we propagated the information given in this book, we'd find, I think, that it would fall more into the ordinary person's scope of understanding. If you knew someone you thought was at risk, I'm sure you would be more inclined to help them if you knew more about the whole process. Most people worry about the smoking habits of persons dear to them; they comment on it, encourage them to stop or cut down, and so on. But if we informed the public about other issues too, we'd probably achieve more preventive work in families. And this is really the best form of prevention.

This leads me to the second point about prevention. People ought to be aware that there are certain crises in life when 'normal' stress has a greater impact than at other times. If we know when those times occur, it can encourage us to take more care of ourselves and others at those times. Throughout the book I have emphasized the role played in learning how to construct healthy body-mind systems by interpersonal relationships. Many of the bad habits we have described are learned patterns taught to the individual by the dominant people in his or her life. If people, both in and out of the medical profession, could see more clearly the impact interpersonal closeness has on these body-mind systems, then we could probably provide better 'emotional cover' at these crisis times. Let me detail some of the life stages I'm talking about.

VULNERABLE LIFE CRISES

Birth to late childhood   The growing child needs to learn to integrate his body-mind patterns with those of his or her environment. As parents we must provide a stable framework in which the necessary experimental learning can take place. The child's emotional life requires the same experimental learning as in doing maths, learning to speak or learning to play an instrument. We could also teach parents to keep an eye on poor body habits, not so much when the child is two or three, but later, when the child goes to school, or around the ages of seven to ten. We must be aware that children express their emotional distress differently from adults; a bed-wetting ten-year-old, a constipated nine-year-old, a seven-year-old unable to cry — they're all telling us something about what's going on 'inside'.

We have to be careful to teach the growing child how to care for him or herself. We as parents must give children time to be upset, tired, weepy or angry, so that they learn to allow themselves the same time. A child who will sleep when he or she is tired, or put on a coat if cold, is a child who is learning to maintain body resistance; he or she is learning healthy self-protection.

Lastly, we must be careful not to let children focus on us

(as adults) too much; we most protect their right as individuals to look after, experiment and form their own body-mind systems. When a child is stressed at school by something we consider minor, we must encourage them to go through the healthy body-mind activities (talking/crying/coping) that will enable them to grow properly, especially in confidence. We must not force our children to be adult too early.

The dangers in this time sequence are the laying down of bad habits which the child will later find difficult to recognize and change.

Adolescence   This is a difficult time in Western or industrialized societies. Social and psychological demands on the growing teenager are often at odds with the pace of his or her own emotional and physical growth. Worse, it is *the* time in life when it's often overwhelmingly fashionable to smoke, drink, indulge in indiscriminate sexual adventures and to cover the resulting internal questioning and turmoil with a glib, bland and cool exterior. Adolescence is also the time when children can easily separate emotionally from their parents, go underground, and lose touch with guiding figures. All too often parents trust to luck that adolescents will make the right kind of contact with others to replace that lost with parents. All too often it isn't made, and instead the teenager encounters loneliness, isolation, emotional sterility and blandness. Often all the teenager can do to cope with these feelings is to try smoking, drinking, casual sex, and so on, the very outlets we know are easily abused, and they may be readily coerced into the kind of bad habits we've been discussing.

We know, too, that cancer-forming habits are laid down in late-adolescence/early adulthood. Consequently we should focus our attention on this period far more than we do. We should provide adolescents with much more detailed and realistic information about the dangers of smoking, drinking, indiscriminate sex, and so on in a balanced, open way. Teach them about personal and sexual hygiene, about how to balance smoking activity with healthy lung exercise. We can teach them a better awareness of their own bodies and we could try to become more aware ourselves of the kinds of problems teenagers undergo. We shouldn't minimize the importance of this stage of growth, and as parents we should try not to abdicate our responsibility to maintain a continuum between the child and the adult. Above all, we should try to maintain contact with our teenagers so that the process of building healthy body-mind relationships doesn't stop at thirteen.

Adulthood   Early to middle adult life is the time when managing a job and interpersonal relationships predominate. Coping patterns, as described in this chapter, can begin to become chronic with the consequences defined earlier. Most of this chapter applies to people in this age group. High-risk young adults are vulnerable to leukaemia, lymphomas and cancers of the reproductive organs. Breast, lung and stomach cancers are the predominant risks overall in this age group, with lung and stomach cancers tending to materialize after forty.

Retirement and old age   The risks in this age group which we could focus on to help prevent cancer are similar to those described in this chapter. In addition, the problems of retirement and loss of partner need special attention. It is a time when we could help people to take better care of themselves. Like the old philosophers, we could encourage older people to explore themselves, their habits and relationships far more than they have ever done. In fact, many retired people wonder how they could have allowed themselves to miss out on proper living in their earlier adult lives; the notion of having a second childhood as you get older is a very real consideration and, I think, a healthy one. Between adolescence and retirement you can get so busy with your job and your family that you have no time for a leisurely consideration of other issues and feelings. We could encourage our old folk to keep fit, to experiment emotionally, to be more self-reliant and so on. There really is no limit to what we can do.

As a society we focus far too much on the links between carcinogens and cancer and not enough on the other factors involved. We should direct some of our energy towards informing people about the links between psychological states and cancer and how seemingly innocuous habits can be related to cancer risk. Secondly, we have focused almost exclusively on cancer in older age groups and our efforts at prevention have concentrated on providing earlier detection, better screening devices and so on. While this is often a matter of medical necessity, cancer begins earlier in life and the most vulnerable age group is the time beteen adolescence and young adulthood. We should direct far more of our efforts towards much earlier prevention and make young adults far more aware of the risks they run than they are at present. Brief messages on cigarette packets are not enough.

CHAPTER 6
Surviving Cancer

We arrive finally at the question of how to survive cancer. When a person actually has cancer the impact of the diagnosis is so enormous, so life-shattering, that it may seem difficult at this point even to think about the role psychology or the mind may have to play in survival. One's first instinct is to shrink in horror from the 'growth' and to want to be rid of it in an immediate and utterly physical sense. Cutting it out, dissolving it, killing it by any physical means possible seem more appropriate concerns than having to consider its existence in any psychological sense. *It* is seen as an alien, an invader, a foreign body or dangerous germ, nothing remotely connected with a state of mind or the practice of bad habits.

These are entirely normal responses, but they are also accompanied by a terror, a helpless fear which, unless one is careful, can cripple the individual's ability to cope with having cancer. What I want to do in this chapter is examine the practical realities of what having cancer means and what being treated for it involves. This will enable us to extend the model used in the book so that the reader is able to create a framework for thinking about his or her own survival. We know that cancer *is* a serious *physical* illness. We know that where it occurs in the body, whether or not it has spread, the stage at which it is diagnosed and whether it can be treated are all factors which help to determine whether or not a person will survive. We know, too, that many of these factors are out of the individual patient's hands. But one vital factor is not, and that is how the individual thinks and feels. This chapter is about how to make the most of the freedom of thought and action remaining to the cancer victim. As I hope you will see, there is a great deal the individual can do.

WHAT HAVING CANCER MEANS

Part of the trouble with developing cancer is that it seems like such a subtle and apparently insidious business. This is especially so for women who may, after many uneventful years, one day feel a lump in a breast, or have cancer detected after a routine cervical smear. It can be such an unexpected shock, like waking up to find that a nightmare is a reality. And the nightmare quality is heightened by the fact that, for the most part, cancer victims feel much the same after they're told as they did the day before the diagnosis. Where is the pain or some other obvious *symbol* of being seriously ill? A high fever, a broken leg, even angina are all, many cancer victims feel, more clear-cut illnesses with definite, identifiable causes and effects. Instead cancer, while being far more serious, usually manifests itself as a relatively small, seemingly insignificant growth; in the case of breast cancer, for example, the size of a pea.

In the early days of knowing one has cancer, the worst thing to face is usually the psychological anxiety or terror of actually 'having cancer'. There is rarely pain or major discomfort. Moreover, this psychological state is accompanied by a series of events that can leave the individual even more bewildered. Let's look at them closely.

Diagnosis   As most people know, cancer is usually diagnosed by a biopsy. This is a minor procedure whereby a sample of the growth is removed from the body and examined by pathologists. These specialists are usually able to tell (a) whether the cells in the sample are benign or cancerous, and (b) if they *are* cancerous, the stage to which the cancer has developed. Diagnosis is done as quickly as possible to avoid unnecessary anxiety for the patient and to allow immediate action to be taken.

Medical action   From the medical point of view, assuming a cancerous growth is in a site which medical technology can reach (either by surgery, drugs or radiation) the sooner that action is initiated the better. There are obvious reasons for this. If, for example, a tumour can be removed in the lung or the breast, this organ can be returned to almost its *status quo* before the growth took place. The growth is stopped by removing it. Prompt action may mean, too, that the cancer doesn't shed cancer cells which might set up in other parts of the body.

At this point in the treatment of cancer these considerations are paramount. The aim of current medical cancer treatment is to stop the cancer from killing. If this cannot be done, the second aim is to buy time, to inflict as much harm to the cancer as possible so as to prolong the patient's life for as long as possible. It is important to understand these considerations because they guide doctors and other medical staff in how they rate priorities for a person with cancer. It is also important to realize that a number of purely medical factors impose limits (or a framework) on how the patient is treated as an individual; he or she is mainly seen at this point as an urgent medical problem.

For a start, the location of the growth can impose problems for the medical team quite as much as its size. A pea-sized growth in the breast is not as immediately life-threatening as the same size growth blocking the throat or, as in a brain tumour, squeezing an artery. A minor growth in an inoperable part of the body presents another complication. Some parts of the body simply can't be operated on because to do so would cause life-threatening damage, cancer notwithstanding. Similarly, bones and organs can block the ability of X-rays to penetrate tumour sites. At a different level, certain body sites are poorly supplied by the blood network, thus making it very difficult for cancer-killing drugs to penetrate them. Another problem is that many of the anti-cancer drugs available are very effective in destroying cancer cells, but en route to the actual growth site they can get diluted or changed by the body's own immune system and lose their effectiveness. In addition, different individuals respond differently to the same drug, thus creating yet another problem to be solved by doctors.

These problems are enormously complicated; inevitably they preoccupy doctors treating cancer patients. Surgeons, to take one example, must consider whether or not they have cut out all the cancer cells. They worry, too, lest they might accidentally spread the cells by the very act of cutting into the body. There is also the issue of how much a surgeon should remove; in the case of breast cancer, for instance, it might be necessary to remove the lymph nodes and muscles under the armpits, just in case secondary growths have formed there. In spite of biopsy reports and X-rays, the surgeon is still partly in the dark until the moment of incision and discovery. Then vital decisions have to be taken very quickly depending on what is found. Similarly, a physician responsible for giving a cancer patient drugs to combat any cells remaining after surgery has to find the right 'mix' and dosage levels for the specific individual and quickly; time lost may allow cancer cells to become active again.

Follow-up medical action   Fast effective action is, by and large, the immediate goal of doctors in a cancer team. In a very short space of time the cancer patient might find him or herself in hospital undergoing surgery, and he or she will wake up feeling distressed and possibly confused. Not all cancers are managed by surgery; radiation, heat treatment and drugs may be used first, but whatever is done will usually be done quickly. It is only after the initial medical onslaught is over that the cancer victim will have the time to take stock of what has happened.

This 'taking stock' is no easy task. Most cancer teams today do not rely on one course of action alone; there are many follow-up activities which again impose on the patient's life. And of course, for the patient, the results of the initial onslaught have still to be lived with — the scars of surgery, the loss of part or all of an organ, the side-effects of X-rays and drugs, and so on. All these have their own impact on the cancer victim's mind.

Knowing what these effects are can be helpful. Most people, after an upset or trauma, want to get back as quickly as possible to normal life; it provides the reassurance, security and comfort they need to begin to come to terms with what has happened. This is not always entirely possible with cancer; it depends on the kind of cancer it is and the treatment administered. In leukaemia, for example, some treatment programmes isolate the patient in an aseptic unit for a time to help the individual's immune system (depressed by cancer-killing drugs) avoid normal germs and infections that might kill. Similarly, certain surgical procedures require subsequent retraining on the part of the patient; for example, with some cancers of the bowel, a stoma or plastic bag is fitted to an entrance in the stomach to replace the removed bowel and closed anus.

As a guiding rule the extent of surgical activity, the frequency and intensity of radiation and the kind of anti-cancer drugs employed are determined by the kind of cancer and stage of its development. In breast cancer, for example, there are three possible operations; simple removal of the tumour lump, removal of sections of the breast, and the more radical procedure of removing the breast, lymph nodes and some muscles under the armpit. Consequently, recovery may be either a complex procedure or relatively minor, depending on the operation undertaken and on the stage of cancer growth. Similarly, in bowel cancer, removal of the bowel and closure of the anus is indicated only in severe cases of cancer; surgical resection of the intestine or bowel is a simpler, less traumatic operation in which the cancerous section of the bowel is cut out and the healthy parts rejoined. Recovery from and adjustment to the latter is very much easier than to the former.

Follow-up radiation treatment and/or the use of drug therapy are to some extent less distressing than surgery, but they carry with them side-effects which can, and often do, cause problems. Hair loss, skin-burning, pain, nausea, vomiting and depression have all been associated with these treatment methods. Cancer is such a powerful process that it requires powerful weapons to reverse its effects; radiation levels have thus to be far higher than normal tolerance allows, and anti-cancer drugs are capable of wreaking severe destruction *en route* through the body to the growth. Most treatment programmes recognize this and limit treatments to specific time spans in order to allow the body to build up strength and recover in between treatments. It is also worth bearing in mind that researchers are constantly searching for more effective drugs with fewer side-effects. Again, the extent of side-effects will depend on the type and spread of cancer: drugs used in treating leukaemia, for example, tend to have greater side-effects than those used in treating cervical cancer.

Lastly, it is also customary for treatment teams to recommend major changes in habits; patients may be advised to stop smoking, change their diet or to take exercise. Of course, how big a part any related habit played in one's life prior to cancer would affect one's ability to cope with the programme.

Change in status   Throughout this time one's reality changes. From being an active part of a family and a community one becomes a patient with the feeling of a possible death sentence pending. Suddenly one is forced into contact with people one doesn't know, machines that can appear frightening and events that are almost entirely out of one's control. It helps to know what effects these experiences can have and how they might affect your treatment.

First on the list, according to research into patients' own experiences, is the sudden loss of contact with the family, especially physical and emotional contact. The 'physical' absence of familiar people in the environment (except for visiting times) frequently results in loneliness. Secondly, people worry about how the family and friends are coping. For many patients these concerns can become obsessive, directing attention away from what is actually happening to them in the hospital.

Next in importance is the effect of suddenly finding oneself dependent on doctors and nurses. This may or may not be a distressing experience, depending, of course, on how skilful medical staff are at providing comfort and support and on how much time they have to do so. In the security of their families, cancer-prone people (as we saw earlier) tend to have well-established ways of getting their needs attended to and coping with stress and upset. Now, suddenly, they are faced in hospital with busy, professional people who may or may not be able to provide the same emotional response. Sometimes the attitudes and behaviour of doctors and nurses can be a source of acute distress on their own, not necessarily through any lack of care on their part, but through the sheer lack of experience the cancer patient may have had with medical staff. This problem, incidentally, is now receiving considerable attention in hospitals and some wards pay special attention to these needs.

Sometimes doctors and other professionals may contribute anxiety through their own feelings as private people; if they are emotionally unable to cope with being depended upon, they feel harassed and distressed by their patients' needs and they respond by being brusque, defensive, cold or aloof. Others may be warm and caring when all is going well and they feel on top of the task, but they may abruptly ignore or avoid a patient's emotional needs if a relapse occurs and they feel they've failed the patient. Other doctors do the reverse and become more caring when problems crop up. The hospital, remember, is a complex psychological world in its own right and the professionals are exposed to the same fears and dreads as ordinary people.

Coping with cancer can be as distressing to a doctor as to his or her patient and this will affect relations between the two. Also bear in mind that till very recently most doctors did not even tell their patients their cancer diagnosis, and psychological aspects of illnesses are only now being generally recognized as important factors in survival. The same goes for the recognition of the right of patients to information about what is happening to them.

I have now described what happens once you are diagnosed as having cancer. It happens all at once and can knock you off your feet, leaving you utterly confused and shocked. So, when the pressures have abated and there is time to think, it is obviously going to be very important that you make the best use of the time available. Let's look now at what you can do.

How To Think About Having Cancer

Many cancer victims when they do finally have a little time to themselves are inclined to do one of two things: first they might concentrate on 'getting by' — on just being 'all right', and reassuring themselves in order to avoid expressing upset. This can take a number of forms, many of them involving the kind of clichéd *blandness* we discussed in Chapter 3. Some people simply trivialize what has happened to them: they reassure themselves with clichés often unwittingly fed to them by medical staff, relatives and other patients: 'Oh, it was only a very small lump' or: 'They took it all out — nothing to worry about. It's back to normal now.' Other people adopt a wan smile or expression and shrug helplessly 'It's all over for me now, just a matter of time,' they might say, giving up both a realistic appraisal of what might happen and all thought of any role they might play in recovery. All these reactions help to repress the terror and fear inside.

Secondly, cancer people might focus their conscious attention on things outside themselves to distract their minds from actively thinking about their circumstances. Thus they might worry about events in the family, about the state of their homes, their gardens, their jobs — all important issues that have to be faced, but not if they are to become obsessions which replace thinking about themselves and their cancer. Cancer people might also willingly discuss their treatment or their reactions to it in impressive detail without actually living through the emotions that should accompany the words. There is evidence too that at least a portion of patients' reaction to treatment and the intensity of their experience of side-effects may be the only way some have of expressing distress. In particular, nausea and vomiting may be in part emotional reactions as much as somatic reactions to the situation. Vomiting and nausea are well-known symptoms of intense fear expressed in a socially or medically approved way. Many patients also develop aversions to anything associated with the hospital; their doctors, hospital smells, injections, and so on; this is a manifestation of fear in much the same way as nausea and vomiting.

Don't misunderstand me here. I'm not trying for a single

moment to minimize the *reality* of all drug side-effects; they are considerable and they can be serious. Worrying about the family and side-effects are key issues in the experiences of the cancer victim that must be attended to, but one must be careful that they don't swamp all available time and outlets of expressing emotions. Let's see what should also be borne in mind alongside these issues.

Finding thinking time   It is vital that the cancer victim be able to create space in his or her day (and in his or her mind) to think about themselves, what has happened and what they are going to do. Just about everything I intend discussing in this chapter requires that the victim have the time to reflect and make plans. Survival partly depends on being able to organize life and body-mind systems to help fight the growth. The sufferer might feel selfish or helpless about doing this, but as you will see, there are many ways of tackling the task.

Thinking about cancer   The key component in what I have to say about surviving cancer centres around the individual's ability to think clearly about what is actually going on and what he or she can do about it. If the cancer victim prefers to think about cancer as something separate from the way he or she functions as a body-mind entity, then they won't, I believe, be making use of all their resources. If you've developed cancer, it is much more useful to think about cancer in the context of the kind of life you led before you knew of its development. If you have followed the model described in this book you'll be aware of what this means.

Start by seeing the growth as the result of the interaction of the habits discussed in Chapter 3. When cancer develops it is, if you like, the body's last-ditch attempt to cope with a situation that it has had to live with for a long time. Like the uncared-for engine in an old car, it has finally developed a crippling problem. The years of (albeit unwitting) misuse and inattention have finally caught up.

Cancer is a sign that the damage done by, say, exposure to carcinogens, can no longer be contained by the body's defensive system. The central nervous system overrides may have been used once too often and the cancer cells which may previously have been held in check overwhelm it and begin to corrupt normal cells. As they spread out they form a mass, which we detect as a lump in a breast, for example, or a swelling in an intestine. Left unattended at this point, cancer cells subvert the immune system even further, coercing the system's local agents into accepting cancer cells as part of the body. Again you can see the force of habit at work; if the local immune centre keeps sending warning or 'help' messages to its support systems (other parts of the immune system, as well as to the central nervous and endocrine systems), but help never arrives, or arrives too late and in too little force (being delayed or diluted, for example, by stress or other preoccupations in the body's networks), it begins to think it's got it all wrong. Since the body doesn't react to the help calls, the local centre gradually gets into the *habit* of not bothering to send out signals; eventually it lets cancer cells pass by into the body unmolested and this is how metastases occur. Once the cancer cells have spread to the local lymph nodes they are in what amounts to a fast lane to wherever else in the body they want to go.

Now think of what happens when a growth is successfully removed before this latter stage happens. The lump is gone, the damage removed and the organ is returned to a normal state, apart from the scar which soon heals anyway. What happens, though, if some cancer cells remain and/or you continue in your old habits exactly as before? That is, if once the scare is over, out come the cigarettes and your emotions go back into cold storage? Clearly, if no cells remain and you return to your old habits, it is entirely possible that the whole process will start up again. If cancer cells remain *and* you return to your old habits, the process may both start up again and accelerate even quicker because of the presence of residual cancer cells in the organ.

If you have radiation treatment or drug therapy these will help to keep the growth under control. But patients can't be kept on drugs for ever and they do have to take breaks to recover, possibly leaving them at risk for that time.

What does this all mean for someone who wants to survive? If a person undergoes treatment for cancer, he or she should also support this treatment by attending to the set of habits that enabled the growth to occur in the first place. Doing this not only helps protect the individual during breaks from treatment, but it removes the conditions which could start the process all over again or encourage the remaining cells to grow. Further, I believe that if the individual's overall psychological and body-mind state can be radically and quickly improved then the risks of metastases diminish and, in all probability, any remaining cells will be eliminated by a rejuvenated and newly-efficient immune system.

These are the issues that cancer victims should tackle as soon as they can. Speed is essential because time may be limited and the behavioural work an individual has to do needs to be almost as quick as any medical treatment. The faster you act, the quicker you help your body to fight your cancer. Which brings me to the last point I want to make in this section

Who survives cancer?   Over the years a considerable body of evidence has accrued about the psychological characteristics associated with people who do survive cancer. Significantly, these findings tie in very comfortably with the model used in this book and with the kind of attitude towards cancer described above.

The most consistent finding emerging from both actual research and clinical experience is that survivors are willing to *fight* cancer. These individuals say to themselves: 'I've had a terrific shock. I want to live and I'm going to drop everything else and make any changes necessary to beat this thing.' Other findings about the psychology of survivors reveal a zest for tackling their problems and a strong will to survive. Survivors offer the following advice, according to one report; 'Stay busy, stay active and get as much information as you can about what's going on.'

A more complex series of investigations performed in various centres have provided us with a deeper view of what actually constitutes the survivors' psychology. According to a British team, while long term survivors tend initially to use denial ('I won't think about it') as a defence from facing up to cancer, they soon take themselves in hand, confront the existence of their cancer and begin actively to fight. An Israeli team noted that this initial denial is best seen as the patient's means of helping him or her focus on getting back to 'normal' at home with the family as quickly as possible, thus presumably allowing time to gather thoughts together and re-establish security before beginning to take stock.

So the evidence points very much in the direction we've been discussing; survivors get their security back as quickly as possible, glean as much information as they can about their condition and then busy themselves fighting their cancer. Having established the value of thinking positively about survival, we can now examine what the actual task of fighting involves.

THE PSYCHOLOGY OF SURVIVAL

It is not entirely accurate to think of surviving cancer as strictly a 'fight'. The term conjures up images of a boxer bashing someone; while developing a feeling like that is an important part of recovery, it is difficult for many people to imagine how they can 'bash' something when (a) it's inside their own bodies, and (b) all the fighting seems to be being done by medical professionals. Cancer patients have to play an inordinately passive role in their treatments and this can deepen the sense of helplessness they already experience.

What we mean by the term 'fighting' in the context of surviving cancer can be elucidated by our model because it defines the areas where the cancer patient goes astray and thus shows us where a sufferer can take the lead.

Much of what was said in the last chapter applies equally to the task of recovering from cancer. The habits which allowed the cancer to develop have to be examined and changed; the psychological framework which supports those habits has to be modified, and the individual's personal relationships altered to facilitate the new learning. The cancer sufferer faces extra tasks — the terror of having cancer and coping with the shock of surgery or other treatments. If we put all these requirements together, the following remedial action can be identified:

1 Building supporting relationships
2 Coping with family, friends and relatives
3 Coping with the shock
4 Coping with body changes
5 Changing bad habits
6 Changing psychological coping patterns
7 Directing your own survival

Next, we'll examine each in turn and spell out what has to be done, how to do it, and how you can get help if you can't manage on your own.

Task 1: Building supporting relationships   Most of the research on cancer survivors has concentrated on the psychological attributes of the survivor — whether he or she 'fights', or gives up and becomes 'helpless'. One other key factor is common to most doctors' clinical experience; the person who is able to form deep personal relationships is more likely to survive than the person who cannot. To my mind, forming a workable personal relationship is the key (all other factors being equal) to survival, and this is one of the reasons why I put it first on the list of survival tasks.

Why are relationships so important? For two reasons: you will recall that one characteristic of high-risk cancer people is their inability to form close interpersonal relationships and that they tend to feel removed or distant from others. It's fair to assume that this lack of contact helps to reinforce (through lack of experience) the individual's inability to express emotions, and this in turn forces them to be dependent on bad body-mind habits for their emotional release. Improving relationships is a step in the right direction towards modifying the whole chain; improve relationships, improve the expression of emotion and this lessens the need to use bad habits excessively. But there is another factor. When you are told you have cancer and when you are exposed to the trauma of, say, surgery, these distressing events create an enormous need inside you for comfort and reassurance. Surgery is a major crisis for anyone, having any serious disease is a major life crisis, and most ordinary people feel, often for the first time, the need to 'regress', to be comforted rather like when they were children. I've seen big, burly *macho* men grateful to have their hands held by virtual strangers while waiting for surgery. I know how grateful I was after a car crash (not that I'm big, burly or *macho*) when another man, also a victim of the crash, held my hand in the ambulance.

So having cancer creates, paradoxically, the socially-approved justification to get the comfort and contact you need as a healthy person anyway. It's there to be taken advantage of, it's natural, expected and, moreover, there are plenty of people around you to help you — if you look.

It is nevertheless important for us to relate this to individual circumstances. For some cancer people, deepening a close relationship can be difficult; sometimes in spite of family closeness the family itself may make demands and create anxieties that can interfere with the cancer victim's need for comfort. A 'stoic' cancer victim for example may be unable to show deep need to the people with whom he or she is closest; this applies especially to adult male victims who, as 'head' of their households, regard it their duty to *give* reassurance and comfort rather than to receive it. While returning home after treatment creates a sense of reassurance by being able to resume a previous role, this doesn't always involve what is needed for survival. One of the biggest tests for my patients was their ability (or lack of ability) to shift from one role to another — from being a 'giver' if you like, to being a 'receiver' of attention.

A 'supporting relationship' will ideally be one in which you feel safe most of the time. You should also receive actual physical comfort in the form of being held, touched, and generally shown you are cared for. Your partner should 'know' you and understand your needs. Most importantly, in an ideal relationship, your partner should allow you to give vent to all your tears, sadness, anger or terror. Lastly, a truly supporting relationship will give you hope for the future, encourage you to believe in yourself and above all, encourage you to make the changes needed to stay alive. This demands a high degree of maturity and development in the partner; a truly supportive partner will grow and evolve with you as you learn to fight cancer.

You must realize that very few people enjoy this ideal kind

of relationship in all its aspects. It is rare to find one single person who is able to perform all these support functions. It is much more likely to be the case that only marginal support is given. I have however spelt out the 'ideal' type to help you know what to aim for. You don't need all these attributes in one person — you can (and should) find parts of them in a number of different people; so long as you know where to look for what you need it doesn't matter how you get it or put it together. The point is, if you want to survive, you'll need a supporting relationship, and it is up to you and those who care about you to see that you get it.

Now, some people may get much of the support they need from the family. I have seen families rally round to help a cancer victim and I've seen husbands and wives so shocked by the presence of cancer in their partners that they become models of comfort and support. However, I have also seen the reverse, so if you can't get help at home, try somewhere else — friends, relatives, or with whomever you feel safe.

Having a religion or other spiritual belief is another possible avenue for help. For some people a faith can make all the psychological difference, especially if this is coupled with personal contact with a priest or other believers. Again, it doesn't matter *what* you believe, or what religion or faith you have; the *contact* and *support* you receive is the vital part. I have even seen people utterly convinced of the power of a herb or, in one case, a mantra, who have been helped by the *force* of their belief more than its substance.

It is important, then, that you focus on building up the contacts you'll need overall. A comforting spouse is fine, but if he or she won't let you cry, you'll either need to work on that, or find someone else who will let you. Similarly, faith in a religion or in a special diet, perhaps, will help you in one sense, but it must be supplemented by other contact to allow you also to express anger, fear, and so on. The danger involved in putting your faith in one single source of support is that you must be sure that it doesn't encourage you to avoid carrying out the very things you should do to survive. For example, an important part of the work I've done has involved teaching people to be *constructively* selfish and occasionally I've found that deeply religious people find this difficult because they have been taught *not* to be selfish. Similarly, there are some practitioners in both orthodox and alternative medicine who advocate single cures or belief-systems about cancer and ignore or minimize other vital aspects of recovery, thus encouraging their patients to do so too.

It seems clear that if you take responsibility for yourself you'll find somewhere along the line — at home, in the hospital or through other contacts — the kind of help you need. Bear in mind that whatever help you get, you must ensure that the components listed earlier are included in your relationship(s). This, of course, might take time; don't worry, just keep what you have to do in mind. Most of what follows will involve these tasks.

Task 2: Coping with family, friends and relatives   The key thing at this point is facing up to your feelings inside. To do this you must radically reassess your existing relationships with those around you. This might seem strange to any reader who doesn't have cancer; after all, it's the cancer victim who needs the attention and here we're discussing what to do about family and friends. But as many cancer victims know, they worry too much about their families first and themselves second. So here's a little discourse on selfishness which should help survivors get their priorities straight.

An aside on selfishness   We are all taught, as we grow up, to think about other people in our personal lives. The media urge us to care about the poor, starving and needy in the world. In fact, part of the overt moral ethic of our society involves being unselfish, giving to others less well off or less able than ourselves, and justly so; the world is a difficult place. It does us no harm to go without and to be unselfish when and where we can.

Similarly, in the family, parents have to be unselfish in their attention to their children and, to a degree, unselfish towards each other. But to what degree should you be unselfish? Where do you draw the line? Or should you be unselfish all the time? Cancer victims inevitably start off with a poor attitude to their own needs, have very little experience of knowing where to draw the line and usually subscribe to the belief that they should be unselfish all the time. They then feel inordinately guilty when they break these rules and later angry or upset for feeling guilty and not getting the attention they need. This builds up into a vicious circle where more unselfishness is practised to compensate for the anger and so on *ad infinitum.*

When one is a child, it is natural to be almost entirely selfish. If a child has a pain, or a need, it is the limit of the child's focus and he or she will wail or nag until the need is attended to. For a normal growing child, this excessive selfishness is gradually balanced with the need to wait, to think about others and their needs, and ultimately leads to the healthy habit of consciously thinking about when and where to be selfish and unselfish. The basis of successful interpersonal relationships as an adult, in fact, demands that a couple be able to think about and discuss their respective selfish needs and to evolve ways of acting on these needs. In a proper relationship, there is no role for pure selfishness or pure unselfishness; there has to be both. Exploring and challenging levels of selfishness should form a vital, ongoing part of the relationship.

If, however, as a child, you have been taught *never* to be selfish, or if your selfish needs have been hammered out of you, you will have evolved a poor attitude towards your own needs. If, further, as is the case with most cancer victims, expressing emotional needs has been banned, ignored or characterized as 'selfish', then real problems can occur. Instead of feeling you have the right to express your emotions or your needs (to learn how to balance something it must first be expressed), you concentrate on avoiding your own feelings and focus on those of others around you. While doing this you may feel resentment, neglected or ignored in your own right. Cancer people feel lonely and isolated because they have been trained to be unselfish about their own emotions, so these feelings remain locked away like a guilty secret.

When it comes to unravelling all this, more problems can emerge and it is as well that you and those around you know what they are. If you block off emotions and punish 'selfish' thoughts, when you do get around to being selfish (as you must if you want to survive), you will not know the first thing about doing it properly. You're almost certain to be either too selfish or too unselfish, or swing violently between the two in the begin-

ning. Please be patient. If you have a good relationship, your
partner will understand. The point is, you have to think about
your own needs and especially about your emotions and bad
habits. You must expect to feel very guilty about your 'selfishness', but push through it.

When I say, therefore, that you have to be able to cope
with your friends and family, I mean that you must care for
them just as you have in the past, but you must also add in time
for yourself. Do it slowly at first and get them used to the idea;
get them used to not disturbing you at set times; lock yourself
away if you must. Then increase the time you devote to yourself.
This is vital — after all, if you want to be truly unselfish, think
of your family in the long run. They'd much rather you
recovered from cancer and are around for as long as possible. If
you want to do that, start off by learning how to be selfish and
self-centred. Now *that's* a good way to be selfish — think of
yourself so that you'll help them.

Task 3: Coping with the shock   Once you are clear about this
you can get on with the kinds of things about which you should
be selfish. At the top of the list come all those feelings about
having cancer and having treatment. You have to let them come
out. And what does that mean? Two things. One, you must
accept them for yourself; that is, you must accept how upset
and distressed you are. It is not natural to be bland or stoical; no
one should cope with shock by suppressing all these feelings.
You can be bland and stoical if you like with strangers or
outsiders but start off by registering the upset to yourself.

Second, you must show what's 'inside' to someone. You
must cry or scream; you must feel sorry for yourself, feel futile,
useless, hostile or angry. Show the pain inside to someone,
anyone — it doesn't matter.

There really is a magic formula for coping with stress;
animals do it — when they've had a fight they show upset, then
run away, lick their wounds (or be licked) and then get back on
their feet again. Don't try to miss steps; it's unnatural.

When a shock is experienced, a person feels more exposed
and more vulnerable than at other times. It is natural to feel
extremely needy, even hungry for comfort. It's natural to want

to regress and be a baby. Having cancer is about the worst shock
a person can experience in life and consequently these natural
emotions are felt more keenly. So what should you expect? What
does a person go through when experiencing shock? These are
not trite questions; many cancer people after a lifetime of
covering up their feelings, are almost as upset by their own
distress as they are about having cancer or even surgery. They
are terrified lest these feelings 'inside' overwhelm them and,
'God forbid,' cause them to break down. It helps, therefore, if a
cancer victim knows what to expect from being shocked, so that
instead of fighting the rising tide of distress, they ride with it and
don't feel so afraid of 'falling apart'.

   The shock reaction chain   The most important part of
being shocked is the experience of *disorientation*, the feeling that
your world has gone out of control, you don't (yet) understand
why, and you don't know what to do. Your conscious mind is
still set on familiar routine, on a set time-sequence of actions
and events. Shock cuts into that massively and grabs your
attention in a completely different direction, which you have
great difficulty in relating to your routine consciousness.

   To cope with this, your mind will usually *freeze* your
emotional reactions to the new information. Some people's
minds shut off so completely that they faint; most go blank or
slow down. The mind, naturally well equipped to handle shock,
isolates your shock reactions for a while, lets you continue
thinking along routine lines, and brings you back time after time
in gradually-increasing exposures to the new reality or direction.
Haven't you ever had an unhappy experience, no matter how
trivial, and found that you 'can't get it out of your mind'?
Images keep popping up uninvited. This is gradual exposure,
gradual adjustment to the event. This is to let you get used to
the *idea* of the shock; to let your mind prepare itself for the next
phase which is *regression*.

   As you think about the shock, your mind begins systematically to let you collapse. We call it letting the shock 'hit' you
little by little; as you think about it, ideas and feelings begin to
well up and your emotions respond by regressing to more childlike, natural forms of coping. Remember, the healthy adult
person, while ordinarily behaving in a very non-regressed,

controlled way, is quite able, even practised, in letting him or herself collapse when necessary. Healthy adults practise these habits with partners and friends; for example the friend with whom you burst into tears, or the partner you rage at. They are the working material on which proper interpersonal intimacy is based.

For its own survival the body demands a collapse into what is known as *constructive regression*. It can cope with the shock only if you let the tears flow, if you can let yourself be comforted, and so on; this defuses the pressure on the body and then the next phase, recovery, can begin. Constructive regression means that you collapse gradually, in the right body-mind ways. It doesn't mean that you collapse into helplessness, or into hyperactivity where you rush around telling everyone how upset you are. Nor does it mean that you should wilt with fatigue and wander around putting on a semi-brave front. Constructive regression means showing *real* emotions, *real* tears, *real* body distress. The better you can cry, the better you can be comforted, the better you can help your body and mind adjust. This means, usually, lots of physical contact, lots of being held, and lots of clinging on to the people you feel safe with. This is the time to be a needy child or even a baby.

Recovery, the next stage of the normal shock experience, is a slow process. Provided the earlier stages have been experienced, the body automatically begins to build itself up for coping. If you cry properly, for example, you defuse the tension inside and this is followed by proper body sleep and proper mind sleep. This in turn enables your body to re-stock properly and your mind to begin (initially in dreams) the process of preparing your consciousness to accept what has happened. When you wake up, you are, as a result, in a better state to move on. Little by little, you'll start planning how to cope, how to re-organize yourself, and so on. As time passes you slowly begin to reverse the regression process until you feel that once again you are on top of what is happening, that you're taking an active and helpful role in your own destiny.

This is the normal person's shock reaction chain and cancer victims should expect (and be encouraged) to go through the same chain, being constructively selfish.

Task 4: Coping with body changes   If you like, think of the shock reaction as falling into two parts, the first part being the normal initial shock we discussed above and the second, the shock associated with having cancer in your body and all that it involves. Included here are the problems of coping with scarring after surgery, and drug and radiation side-effects. Research has shown that many patients experience depression, sexual difficulties and anxiety in the months (and years) following treatment, nearly all of which arise as a result of having to cope with changed body states.

The loss of an organ or part of an organ is a traumatic experience on its own. When accompanied by the knowledge that the loss was caused by cancer, the trauma is likely to be intensified, depending to some extent on the way the organ was regarded beforehand. People suffering from breast or cervical cancer necessitating relatively radical surgery or radiation treatment, and those where a stoma (the plastic bag used to collect body waste) is fitted after closure of the bowel, are most vulnerable to the experience of changed body state. We will look briefly at the psychological problems peculiar to each and at the help you can be given.

Breast and cervical cancer   A great deal has been written about the reactions women experience to these cancers and it is well worthwhile reading up about how other people have coped. In a number of hospitals groups of women meet to share these experiences, and research reports have suggested that these can be very helpful. However, some people do not like group experiences and manage well enough on their own. It's a matter of choice.

The main psychological problems stem from how the person feels about the change to the organ. In breast cancer, the damage is external and obvious. In cervical cancer, it is internal and not, of course, obvious. Two key emotions are involved; the reaction to being disfigured, and anxiety about what this might mean to a woman's personal and sexual relationship.

Feeling disfigured can result in a person experiencing intense feelings of self-pity and later, revulsion. For many women who have had radical breast surgery, it is months before they can face touching or looking at their scars, let alone allow anyone else (even a partner) to do so. This is a very natural reaction, and provided the scar is cared for and its healing takes place properly, it is nothing to worry about. In time, with patience and care, most people can slowly come to terms with the physical reality of surgery. Having someone around to help you go through this stage is a tremendous source of reassurance and forms an important part of making a healthy adjustment.

Keeping the feelings of ugliness and revulsion to yourself can cause intense distress. In my experience it is very important that an individual get to the basic, underlying distress and tackle that rather than focus excessively on the scar or the physical loss of the breast. Most of my patients needed reassuring at a very simple level that the loss of the breast and/ or the scar did not mean the loss of 'identity' as an individual. At a 'baby' level, I felt they were asking whether the loss of this social fetish harmed or changed them as people.

At a rational level, the answer is, of course, that nothing should really change. Loss of a breast isn't loss of a life, neither should it connote loss of status. Mutilation and loss can be adjusted to both by the victim and by her partner, provided the problems of revulsion and readjustment are dealt with. There is now considerable evidence to show that the psychological trauma of breast cancer can be alleviated when both the victim and her partner come to grips with the fact that they both feel distressed and repulsed by what's happened. Repulsion is natural provided it is (a) recognized and admitted to, and (b) worked on. Let me describe the case of a couple I saw, Bob and Rita.

Rita was referred to me by her GP as suffering from depression eighteen months after being operated on for breast cancer. When I first saw her it was clear that while she put on a brave front she was in despair, not so much over the operation but that she would lose her relationship with her boyfriend, Bob. After a few interviews I asked to see them together because I felt that a few clarifying words might help them at least tackle what I thought was their central problem. Both had coped bravely and tenderly with each other after Rita's operation but neither had coped with the distress each had felt as a result of it. On Bob's part he seemed slowly to have lost interest in making love, and while remaining close and appearing responsive, he'd given

Rita the impression that his mind was elsewhere.

To cut a long story short, this proved to be the case. Bob chatted to me over the next few weeks and was very relieved to find that he wasn't 'being a heel' by avoiding love-making because he couldn't bear to touch Rita's scar. Once brought out into the open, he was able to relive some of the anguish and revulsion he felt towards Rita after surgery and to explore the intense guilt he felt about this. What I did was just to let him talk and trusted that his underlying love for Rita would emerge once his anxiety had worked its way out. I didn't, at this stage, encourage him to discuss his feelings with Rita because she was troubled enough as it was. Just having a willing ear, however, helped Bob and he welcomed the opportunity to tackle his emotional neglect of Rita. Rita in turn felt more sure of Bob, felt he was being more honest and together they began to relive the events of the previous eighteen months. Eventually they were able to talk about their true feelings and for the first time look at the breast and the scar to see what it was that they were avoiding.

With Bob and Rita, once they learnt to trust each other and talk openly, they soon saw that covering up revulsion with polite and caring clichés caused far more distress than the actual cancer. If you hide a revulsion from yourself and your partner, you freeze the feeling inside; unexpressed, it can't go anywhere. Unfreeze it and you can begin to explore the realities of the situation. Most revulsions are caused by primitive fears, formless bits of terror that should be seen for what they are; baby terrors that need baby comfort. To cover them up is to give them a status they don't deserve. Cancer is distressing, having surgery or radiation is unpleasant, but once it's over not a lot has really changed. As I said to Bob; 'What's a scar between friends? She's still the same person in every other way, will make love in the same way, breathe the same, think the same. You've been fixated on the scar because you've not explored how upset you've been. Get upset and let her get upset and you'll soon see that the scar is nothing, that what's come between you is blocked emotions. You've also got to face the fact that your own problems have helped to block Rita's recovery. Don't just see it as her problem.'

The key element in my treatment was to get them over this fixation on the scar. Their blocked emotions had led them to politely ignore the breast, to leave it out of their love-making and their discussions. Opening up the issues took some of the weight away from the scar, but to be really effective, this had to be backed up with actual behaviour change. I encouraged them to touch the scar, to make love again as if nothing had changed. This simple act provided the real proof — that the scar was irrelevant. Incorporating the scar into their normal initiate behaviour combined with expressing the emotions previously linked to the scar in their proper context did more than just improve their relationship. As I outlined earlier, it is entirely possible that cancer in the breast may well be set up by poor acceptance and use of the breast and by corresponding hormonal deficiencies associated with conflicting emotional attitudes to the organ. After surgery and healing have taken place, it seems to me vital that the breast be not only used properly, but pre-existing problems associated with the personality of the cancer victim be explored and resolved. Rita had had such problems, and with her confidence restored and proper use made of the breast, she was able to work on those. I was able to get her and Bob to see that recovery demanded that these pre-existing problems (and pre-existing problems in their relationship) be the main focus of attention. In time they could see that the scar and the difficulties it had caused was a very minor issue compared to what really needed to be done.

Not everyone is able to recognize, let alone work on, these feelings, but if you can use someone to help you over this time, it will definitely enable you to survive better. Ultimately a cancer victim has to face what has happened. Facing it by going through the emotions outlined here will ensure that you are helping your body to cope. If you find that you're slipping into depression, becoming more and more isolated and lonely, if you or your partner are gradually withdrawing from intimacy with each other — try to do something about it. Get help when and where you can.

Coping with a stoma   Having a plastic bag fitted to your stomach is about the most radical result of cancer surgery there is and the changes involved are considerable. Like breast and cervical cancers, apart from the shock of the diagnosis and surgery, there are the problems of depression and coping with intimacy. Many people report 'intimacy' problems, clinically defined as sexual worries and worrying about what other people think of them.

The first and immediate consequence to face is the horror of having to think about evacuating your bowels through a hole in your side. Fortunately, if you have to do it every day, you quickly adjust; indeed, a person I know who has had a stoma for seventeen years now says, 'It's quicker, cleaner and less trouble than going to the toilet ever was.' However, I know she needed a lot of support in the first few years and was helped by her doctors who patiently listened to her and gave her tranquillizers from time to time to help her adjust to what had happened. She was helped, too, by the fact that she underwent her operation late in life and after her husband died:

'I could cope with it, I realized, if I didn't have to share a bed with someone. Since my husband had died and I was nearly sixty, I made a conscious decision to give up men. I realize I might have been avoiding things there but, what the hell, I wanted to enjoy my old age and to survive cancer. This was my way.'

Why I've quoted her here is not to recommend her decision for everyone else, but to show that she took her own decision to look after herself; she got rid of her current 'boyfriend', moved in with a sister and took her comforts from the companionship of animals and friends. What mattered was that after the initial shock she faced up to what she wanted (or needed) to do.

Other people organize their lives around their stoma. Again, provided the correct emotional experiences are gone through, then wonders of adjustment can be performed, as Albert, a fifty-eight-year-old cancer survivor notes:

'The wife and I were in a pretty rough state for two years after my op. Nothing said, nothing done, but it was bad. I hated myself for having this bloody bag in my guts and I just didn't want to even look at it, let alone let her see it. But one night we had a bit too much to drink and I suppose she felt a bit, you know, randy, and I got tense, but she suddenly took over and for the first time in my life I was made love to. From then on we did it every now and again, a bit furtive you know, but gradually we realized that it wasn't the end of the world. You can work round it, you know.'

They still don't talk about it, have never, in fact, gone over their problems, but they nevertheless learned to live together better. Albert no longer feels useless and no longer thinks his life is over.

The key thing here is to be able to work around the problems and to pick up the pieces of your life as before. Giving in to the difficulties and the shock for too long and losing your ability to think about helping yourself (or, as often happens, allowing yourself to be helped by someone), does the emotional damage in the long run. As I said earlier, there is a right and wrong way to be upset. Expressing the feelings of distress, self-hate or ugliness, and then 'collapsing' are the main feelings that should be shown in the beginning, or over the first few months after surgery or other treatment. Thereafter it's important to combine being upset with coming to terms with what you have to do to get on with the rest of your life.

It is a good idea to obtain some idea of the role anger may play in the months after surgery or other treatment; this can help you and those around you to manage a great deal more easily.

An aside on anger and hostility   When a person's body lets him or her down, or becomes scarred or 'ugly', one reaction to the new situation is to feel angry and bitter. This applies especially to cancer people; many feel that they don't deserve it and others feel that they have not enjoyed life properly beforehand or not lived enough for themselves. Initially this mixture of hostility, sadness and intense self-pity can turn into irritability with other people. Sometimes unexpected outbursts of anger will be directed at those closest to the person. It can cause the cancer victim to feel intense guilt, which results in the individual trying very hard to express no emotions at all, which in turn can lead to an intense feeling of internal pressure. Then, when quite ordinary things go wrong — a door slams, a glass breaks, a screw-top jar won't open — the pressure can become unbearable.

At these times, family and friends can be most helpful. If

they understand that being irritable and tense is the only way
some people can express their upset, and that they still need to
be loved or accepted whatever form their hostility takes, then
this will help them get through this period. One of the biggest
tasks psychotherapists, doctors and nurses face in coping with
patients experiencing intense distress is learning not to take the
patient's anger or hostility personally, not to withdraw from
them and not to become hostile in turn. If you can show them
that you *sympathize* with their distress and that you're capable
of ignoring or *overlooking* their irritability or bad temper, you're
showing them that you *care* for what they're going through.
Holding them, or being kind when they're feeling guilty, and
perhaps discussing their feelings can further help them to
appreciate that you are aware of what's going on. Again, if you
are a friend or relative of a cancer victim and need help at this
level, seek it from a professional — someone with experience in
cancer or crisis management. Similarly, if you are a cancer
victim and want to learn how to express yourself more comfortably, seeing a good psychotherapist, social worker, GP or nurse,
can be invaluable.

   Coping with anti-cancer medication   A last source of
body-change to concern us in this section is how to cope with the
side-effects of anti-cancer medication. For a long time, cancer
victims were left alone to battle with the sometimes quite
severely debilitating effects of cancer drugs. These include loss
of hair, burning and skin pain, nausea, vomiting, constipation
and diarrhoea. Certain cancer drugs are now also known to
cause more depression in patients than other drugs, on top of
any existing emotional distress.

   Fortunately, these hazards are now in the process of being
remedied; researchers have developed drugs with fewer side-
effects, and psychologists and psychotherapists have investigated methods of helping people to cope better with the effects.
Patients in a number of cancer units are now taught a variety of
psychological devices to minimize their symptoms and are being
given much more support for their problems than in the past. If
you have these difficulties, don't just struggle bravely on — ask
your doctor for help.

Task 5: Changing bad habits   It goes without saying that this, together with the next task, constitute the major survival tasks. All that has gone before is aimed at getting you to the point where you can change the very behavioural and psychological patterns that contributed to the cancer risk in the first place. This, if you like, is where the fight really begins.

If you want to survive you will have to take a good look at your risk patterns as outlined in the previous chapters and then to modify them so that your body is able to help the surgeons, physicians and radiologists to combat any cancer cells remaining inside your body.

Strange as it may sound, far too many cancer victims do *not* give up their bad habits after knowing they have, or have had, cancer. I have known smokers take up smoking again once they have been reassured that there is no trace of lung cancer left. In fact, I have even noted a certain bravado about this: 'See, even cancer couldn't make me stop.' Part of the problem, I appreciate, is that not enough direction is given in this area; most people are aware of the associations between smoking and lung cancer, but not everyone is familiar with the links between their habits and other cancer sites. After working your way through this book, you should have no trouble appreciating the urgency of making changes.

The major concern here is to improve your overall health. Apart from any bad habits you might have (which we'll come to in a moment), it is vital that you review just about everything you do to ensure that wherever possible you are working at your health. Begin by running through the following list of guide lines, organized around the basic actions of the body.

Breathing   Make sure the lungs get plenty of fresh air and that they are regularly and routinely exercised. Remember, whether or not a person has (or has had) lung cancer, smoking is a treble hazard to anyone suffering from any form of cancer. It is a hazard first of all to allow carcinogens into the body. Secondly it is a hazard to anyone whose general immune system is lowered, and remember, cancer victims nearly always experience psychological and emotional shock which lowers resistance and makes them especially vulnerable. Thirdly, and most important, anti-cancer medication is often accompanied by effects which act to depress the functioning of the cancer person's immune system. As noted earlier, in order to help the cancer drugs arrive at the cancer-site intact, the body's immune responses often have to be lowered so that they do not interfere with the medication. While this is happening, the individual may be extremely vulnerable to the effects of a variety of foreign subtances he or she would ordinarily manage. Adding cigarette smoke to this list is little short of suicide.

If you can't stop smoking, seek help. It is absolutely essential that you do not mess around with your body at this stage and professional assistance might be vital. You may not get a second chance.

Breathing is an important thing to think about even for people who don't smoke. The lungs, like every other part of the body, need to be taken care of. Focusing on breathing properly, actively avoiding public or private places where one might be exposed to smoke, fumes or other irritants, is a good way of learning how to be properly selfish or self-caring. Knowing you have cancer should serve as an incentive; it is your right to look after yourself and if this means avoiding smoky rooms, then do so. Take the necessary steps even if it means asking your husband, wife, mother or father not to smoke in your presence. If they won't co-operate, don't just wilt and give in. This is an important first step to take in being constructively selfish; teach people to *think* about your needs by teaching yourself how to think about them. Fight for your own clean breathing space.

Eating and drinking   A great deal has been written about diets and cancer and I am certainly not qualified to comment on the value of this literature or on any particular diet. This is a subject about which each individual must make up his or her own mind. However, one thing is clear: eating healthy foods and eating *in a healthy way* are tremendously important for the cancer victim. For one thing, a healthy diet provides the necessary replacement energy, salts and protein to help the victim cope with the emotional shock and the body shock of surgery, radiation or drugs. Specific diets are required to help the body cope with the specific effects of medical treatment, and it is vital that the recommendations of doctors and dieticians be followed. It is no good thinking that you can go straight back to your old eating habits after treatment either: many people not only do not eat enough of the right food, but the *way* they eat contributes to their risks too. I'm thinking here of over-eating or under-eating, eating too fast, excessive use of alcohol, excessive sugar intake, excessive anxiety associated with eating, and so on. Again, this presents an opportunity for the individual to learn how to care for him or herself better. Let me introduce you to Gwen.

Gwen was a thirty-eight-year-old woman who had had a breast removed and was making a good recovery and a good adjustment to her condition but with one problem. She was advised by her doctors to change her diet, but had faced problems when she tried to stick to her cancer diet at home. 'There's just too much pressure. My husband expects his food just like always, my kids hate the idea of dieting, and then there's my mother, whom we eat with twice a week; if I don't eat her food she sulks. So what do I do? I've explained that I have to diet but no one takes any notice; they've forgotten I've had cancer.'

Gwen didn't have the time to cook two sets of meals every day and so she was very quickly coerced into eating as she had always done, just to keep her family happy. This is a classic case of what I am talking about; Gwen had to be helped to *fight* her family properly, to learn how to stand up for herself and to protect herself. Moreover she had to do all this without being too drastic either, which would have caused her more anxiety than she could manage. So with my support she involved her husband and kids in sharing the cooking, let them eat what they wanted and stuck to her diet. The only person who really was 'bloody-minded' was Gwen's mother, who refused to speak to her for two weeks after Gwen arrived to supper bringing her own food with her. With patience and encouragement though, Gwen was able to explain to her mother how vital it was for her recovery, and in doing this Gwen learned to be more forceful and more assertive, which incidentally helped her in other areas too.

Evacuation of waste   The same principles apply when it comes to going to the toilet. A healthy body requires trouble-free and daily evacuation, and a combination of a healthy diet and exercise. Taking the time to relax when you're 'on the loo' is necessary to ensure that this part of your body functions properly. Again, it is essential not to neglect this. Psychological treatment to help people relax, coupled with care and consideration from others in the family, can work wonders. Don't put it off.

Sleeping   Whatever you may feel about the value of sleep, your body and your mind need it. If you are troubled by insomnia or bad dreams, or if you sleep too lightly (malsomnia), seek advice. Apart from the fact that your body needs the rest, your mind's ability to cope with the stresses of having cancer depends on having proper dream sleep, which is indicated by rapid eye movement (REM sleep). This means that you must aim for approximately eight hours sleep per night: four hours is needed by the body, and two to four hours for your mind to dream. It is in dream-sleep that the mind works over the shocks and upsets to the system enabling the individual to adjust.

Exercise   With some exceptions (for example, bone cancers), exercise should form a central part of your life. It helps keep your body and muscles supple, provides stamina and keeps weight down. Consult your doctor about the form of exercise you should take and be sure you do it. Remember, there are all sorts of exercises to cope with just about everyone's needs and every possible complication, so there's no real excuse not to exercise. Again, making time to exercise is a good experience for the cancer victim; it requires learning self-discipline, selfishness and self-assertion. It may also help the individual discover hidden talents, enjoyments and unknown pleasure in social contacts, all of which can be used to help in the fight to survive cancer.

Other body activities   Everything you do, from brushing your teeth to brushing your hair, should now be done with care and consideration. Cancer victims must learn to appreciate that their bodies have to be looked after in every way. One important area in particular is in love-making. Be sure that you don't allow yourself to be hurt or irritated, and also ensure you are scrupulously clean. I appreciate that this can be a very awkward area in which to assert your rights, but it must be done. Take whatever steps are necessary to protect yourself.

Task 6: Changing psychological coping patterns   As an individual changes personal habits, so too does the body-mind network change. The 'fight' in cancer survival is essentially an internal struggle between the old, bad habits and the psychological framework that holds them in place, and the new, healthier habits. The 'fight' emerges and is experienced subjectively as the internal pressure mounts over *not* to be 'selfish', or to give in to social or family pressure and conform. It is also felt as the desire *not* to use the healthy new habits, to take the easy way out and opt for the older, more familiar bad habit. After all, smoking or eating a meal you didn't want, or giving in meekly to someone else's whim, all have their immediate rewards — that momentary relief of the tension inside. Familiarity, the avoidance of conflict, and so on, are very powerful motivators for returning to the pre-cancer *status quo*; while changing your lifestyle — on the healthy side — appears at times to offer very little reward.

It is at this point that the confidence and will of cancer victims to survive can begin to fade, leaving the would-be survivor at his or her lowest ebb. Some people really try hard, begin to look after themselves, change their habits, and then simply give up; the effort of making the changes seems too much and they slide back into their old ways.

The point is this: at the vulnerable time the new habits are still only beginning to be experienced. The individual has had no time to build up a corresponding psychological and emotional framework to support the new learning. The possibility of living better, longer and more healthily is just that — a vague possibility, hovering somewhere in the future. In fact, making the kind of changes I've outlined in this chapter may by now have caused the cancer sufferer to feel a good deal more miserable, more guilty, more tense even — maybe more aware than ever of how much remains unresolved within. And some people believe that cancer victims shouldn't be made to feel these things, that they should be left to die in peace.

These are very sensitive issues. In cases where the diagnosis is hopeless, the cancer widespread and, of course, where intense or chronic pain is a daily feature of the victim's life, then clearly a different approach must be adopted. Improving the quality of life in those cases is extremely important, as is preserving the *status quo* in family life. Cancer spreads its effects beyond the immediate victim and like all serious diseases can psychologically and emotionally scar others in the family. It is as well in these cases to leave things be.

Where chances of survival are very good, however, it's quite a different story. Ultimately though, it is a matter of individual choice.

How can you keep going when it is too soon to know what it feels like to be properly healthy, when it is too soon to experience any of the positive effects of dropping unhealthy habits? This is the stage when having faith, having confidence in your doctors, having belief in anything, counts; when any little breath of hope must be clung to for dear life. To help you get through this stage, it's as well to know something about the psychology of hope and how to make use of it. Building up hope helps the individual build up the psychological patience needed to allow new habits to become established.

The psychology of hope   Having hope is not just a matter of trusting in fate, God, luck, astrology or any other talisman. It involves all those things, but it is much more. It is a psychological framework which can make the difference between surviving and not. At root it means being able to find any one thing which, when thought of, alleviates the feeling of hopelessness, no matter how little. If you like, it is finding something to live for, to cling to, something that is precious or pleasant.

Most of what has been written about hope and symbols of hope has stressed the altruistic or rationally acceptable forms hope can take: religious faith, transcendental belief, love, and so on. But when it comes to sheer survival, it is best to think of hope in the shape of anything that helps an individual. And it is often the case that this takes the form of some childlike, or regressed, thought.

At the Simonton's clinic in Texas, for instance, patients have been helped build up their hope — their ability to hang on — by encouraging them to use any image at all that makes them feel they are coping. Such images might seem infantile to outsiders (imagining the white blood cells in the body chewing up cancer cells like a shark, for example), but they are like a lifebelt to a drowning person.

'Imagining', in fact, is a technique much employed now by certain psychologists, behaviour therapists and cognitive behaviourists. Very simply put, it involves teaching a person how to use thinking about 'nice' or 'safe' thoughts (no matter how childlike) to balance fearful or anxiety-provoking thoughts and feelings. Like repeating a prayer, they serve as mental reassurances and can be used for a wide range of purposes. These techniques are quite easily taught, so do consider using them if you feel your courage waning and have nothing else or no one else to turn to. Nevertheless, they should only be seen as devices to serve you while you begin to reconstruct your psychological life, not as ends in themselves — as 'cure-alls' — because the real end product is improving your own ability to survive. This, remember, means changing habits and your body-mind network sufficiently, so that survival becomes a real possibility.

So assuming an individual has enough hope to keep going, what then? The act of changing habits will on its own have created a certain degree of inner turmoil and anxiety and it is crucial that these anxieties and emotions be attended to in a healthier way. Take giving up smoking, or the anxiety created by a victim being more 'selfish'. For most people, the acts of smoking, being altruistic or unselfish, helped to express or pacify fear or anxiety. Now, without being able to smoke, what do you do with the feelings inside? They don't just go away. Correctly, they should serve as the impetus you need to change your psychological and emotional framework. Face the anxiety inside, face the fact that how you managed in the past was psychologically humiliating and emotionally harmful. Face the fact, too, that you probably did yourself a great deal of somatic harm by resolving these anxieties in ways that caused you to override somatic discomfort, pain and weariness. If you like, and if it helps, get angry with yourself for every time you didn't stand up for your own emotional or psychological rights and try to see that over the years it was every such instance that contributed to the growth of the cancer inside you. Finding new and better ways of reducing your anxiety, being emotional, being creative, can save your life.

Experiencing all these feelings should provide you with the

necessary impetus to restructure your emotional life. You should use them to change the psychological framework in which you live, in which you see yourself. Making these changes constitutes the last step on the road to survival.

Task 7: Directing your own survival   I am not able to give extensive details here about how this last step can be taken; cancer patients are unique individuals who must of necessity tackle this uniqueness in their own way. If I were to detail some psychological and emotional changes, they would not account for others and may even be confusing: one person's meat is another's poison. What I can do, though, is make the following points about how to direct your own survival.

The importance of relationships   Throughout the book you will have noticed how much emphasis I put on relationships. This is because practically all we learn is within the context of relationships. Having people around us provides us all with basic psychological comfort like nothing else can. But there are many different types of relationships. Some can harm us, some can be useful. The point is that if you want to survive, examine your existing relationships carefully. If you can change them (or develop them) to help you cope with being a healthier person than before, i.e. being more open emotionally, more expressive and more demanding, so much the better. But if you can't, don't be afraid to find others who can help you. I'm not talking about having an affair (although that is a possibility for some), or indeed even about sexual relationships; a relationship with a friend, a relative, a doctor, a priest — with anyone, in fact, who can help you achieve a healthier level of psychological functioning. Psychotherapy, for example, is basically a relationship and a potentially valuable one. It, after all, focuses (or should) on making just the changes we're after.

By the same token, if you can't find a suitable relationship, or if you want to work at it on your own, go ahead. This is especially useful in cases where a person is quite unable to behave differently from before at home. Being alone, thinking, reading, trying out new things can all be done without showing anyone else if you don't want to. In fact, I've often taught patients to go off on their own, to cry alone, to cry with a pet, even just to cry with a cuddly teddy bear — whatever works. Similarly, I've encouraged patients to learn how to scream and shout, relax, avoid constipation — all in isolation if necessary. Take your own responsibility. If you've got the determination, you'll find a way to survive.

Learning to be emotional   Above all, as you direct your survival, focus on changing your patterns of emotional expression. Stop being self-destructive and start taking better care of your body by letting the emotions out. Remember, 'inside' you are stuck at the level of a child or an adolescent; like a child or adolescent you'll have to learn how to be emotional. You'll have to act out, make mistakes, and yet not take too seriously the silliness, guilt and anxiety you'll feel as you do so. Crying, being comforted, being happy, sad, upset, depressed, angry — these are normal, proper human emotions that must be felt and expressed. It's your *right* as a person to learn how. Moreover, doing it will help your body and your cancer. The more you do it, the more you will be controlling your own survival.

EPILOGUE
Final Word

What I've tried to do in this book is present a much broader view of cancer and its treatment than most people are used to. I've called it the psychology of cancer because that term helps to get across the idea that the kind of personality, the kind of emotions you have and the way you behave are linked to cancer. What we have been talking about of course is the human organism in its entirety, trying to link the many levels of function of the body together. We have attempted to relate what happens to cell tissue to how the body's neural, endocrine and immune systems interact and we have seen something in turn of how these can be shaped by the way a person lives or behaves.

Above all the main concern has been to show where the individual person fits into the cancer-producing process and where and how he or she can act to avoid getting cancer. I hope by now you will agree that we can no longer afford to think of cancer as a phenomenon that strikes out of the blue in the same way that malaria or smallpox might — through exposure to a single harmful entity. Cancer is intimately involved with how people live — with the kind of choices they make. People are free to smoke, make love, eat, drink and generally behave however they like. What I hope is now clear is that how the individual makes these choices and how he or she carries them out can expose them to cancer risks. What I have set out to do in this book is to spell out in some detail just what these choices imply and how the risks can accumulate. The aim, ultimately, is that you will use this knowledge to good effect, that what you have read will encourage you to start looking at your own habits, your thinking and how you approach difficult problems in life. I firmly believe that armed with enhanced awareness people can cut their cancer risks considerably. Moreover if we think ahead and take steps to protect our children and adolescents by encouraging them to think defensively about cancer, we could begin to envisage the day when cancer would once again be a rare disease.

I hope too that this presentation of what contemporary psychology and psychiatry and related disciplines like psycho-neuroimmunology can do will encourage people to make greater use of the expertise available. Cancer is a major health hazard and it seems to me that mental health professionals should be much more involved than they are at present in prevention and treatment. Further, we as a society should try to overcome our prejudices about seeking psychological help. Not just in the sense of removing the stigma attached to seeing a psychiatrist or psychologist but in the deeper sense of devoting more time to ourselves and our own mental states. In the long run, creating more time to think, to reflect on how we as a society and as individual people are involved in the cancer process, will save lives.

BIBLIOGRAPHY AND READING NOTES

These notes are designed to give the reader some idea of the available evidence around which each chapter was built. Since much of this is technical I have also tried at the same time to make general reading suggestions of a less technical nature to enable the interested layperson to obtain a grasp of the subject.

There are a large number of texts now available for the layperson which provide an introduction to ideas about cancer and its treatment. I found Bodley Scott (1981) and Rosenbaum (1983) useful in this respect, but there are many others of equal value. I don't, incidentally, think the layperson should be put off by technical writings; often a good medical dictionary can help you understand the gist of things, and once you've stopped being intimidated by medical jargon, you'll be surprised how much you'll be able to understand.

INTRODUCTION

Even thirty-odd years on, the best reviews of the role played by psychological or mental factors in the history of medical understanding of cancer are LeShan (1959) and Kowal (1955). Le Shan's is easy to read and has some fascinating quotations from early writers. Look out especially for Gendron (1701) and Burrows (1783). Both reviews also give a fair picture of the way thinking about cancer by psychiatrists and psychologists developed earlier in this century.

CHAPTER 1 UNDERSTANDING CANCER

An interesting insight into how the attitudes of doctors and other professionals to their cancer patients has changed in recent years is contained in two reports; Oken (1961) and Novack et. al. (1979).

For the descriptions and definitions of tumours and growths I have relied on Morehead (1965) and Walter & Israel (1979). Despite its weight and erudition, the latter text is very easy to read. For more up-to-date reviews of what scientists think occurs in cell tissue during malignant changes see Alberts (1983), Berkman & Syme (1979), Berridge (1985), Land, Pavada & Weinberg (1983), Logan & Cairns (1982) Robertson (1983a, b), Snyder (1985), Tabin et. al. (1982) & Weinberg (1983). I recognize that this is perhaps the most controversial and crucial area of contemporary cancer research, and so I have tried to present a formulation that most researchers would roughly agree with.

For the section on what causes cancer I drew on the following: Barker (1984), Barker & Rose (1976), Bodley Scott (1981), Doll (1972), Doll & Peto (1981), Duff & Hollingshead (1968), Fraumeni (1975), Harnden (1983), Kelley (1983), Lips et. al. (1982), Osmond et. al. (1983), Rather (1978), Rubens & Knight (1980) & Whelan (1980).

Polakoff & Rosenbaum (1983) provide a layperson's guide to environmental and occupational cancer risks.

Some readers might be interested in the incidence of some of the cancers mentioned in the text. The following is a selection of articles that might prove informative: Ames (1983), Beresford (1983), Blot et. al. (1983), Hill et. al. (1983), Keller (1983), Klauber (1978), Liddell (1973), McIntyre (1979), Najem &

Molteni (1983), Palmer & Scott (1981), Reif (1983), Stemhagen et. al. (1983), Stocks & Davies (1960), Swerdlow (1983), Taylor (1984) & Wilkins, Reiches & Kruse (1979).

Most basic medical or psychophysiology textbooks will contain information on the structure and function of the Central Nervous, Endocrine and Immune systems. More detailed texts on how the body's main controlling and regulating systems inter-relate with one another are harder to come by and are usually highly technical. An excellent source book for this area with particular emphasis on interactions between the three systems is Ader (1981). See also the following; Ader (1980, 1983a, b), Antonovsky (1980), Bartrop (1979), Bovbjberg, Cohen & Ader (1982), Cassel (1976), Engel (1977), Fabris & Garaci (1983), Mason (1976), Jemmott & Locke (1984), Macek (1982), Stoll (1979) & Tonegawa (1985). This is a brief sample of the growing literature in this area. An excellent and indispensible review, incidentally, of the very new work on linking psycho-social factors to immune functioning is Jemmott & Locke's paper.

Much interest in recent time has also focused on the role played by peptides in providing links between the three systems. Psychologists and psychiatrists have concentrated naturally on brain peptides but there is considerable evidence that local peptides may serve similar functions throughout the body. For an insight into some of this research see Bloom & Polak (1981), Gregory (1982), Katzenellenbogen (1980), Krieger (1983), Polak & Bloom (1982), Polak & Van Noorden (1983) & Snyder (1984).

CHAPTER 2   CANCER AND PERSONALITY

There is as yet no adequate review of this field for the layperson but Cooper (1982), Locke (1983) and Murray (1980) go some way toward filling this gap. The Locke article is written particularly for the layperson.

I used a fairly broad cross-section of research reports to write this chapter. Amongst those I found useful were the following; Achte & Pakaslahti (1981), Apfel (1982), Bahnson (1981), Bahnson & Bahnson (1969), Crisp (1970), Goldberg & Tull (1983), Holland (1981a, b), Holland & Frei (1978), Jacobs

& Charles (1980), Klein (1971), Krasnoff (1959), Lermer (1982), Levine, Silberfarb & Lipowski (1978), McKegney (1979), Miller, Ross & Cohen (1982), Miller & Spratt (1979), Morris et. al. (1981), Moss (1973), Plumb & Holland (1977), Rabkin & Struening (1976), Totman (1979) & Trillin (1981).

The retrospective studies performed in Scotland on lung cancer victims were reported by Kissen (1963, 1967). See also Abse et. al. (1974). The American study on cervical cancer was reported in Schmale & Iker (1966). Le Shan's work is contained in Le Shan (1959, 1966, 1984). The studies performed in London on breast cancer patients come from the Faith Courtauld unit for Human Studies in Cancer, Kings College Hospital — see the articles by Greer & Morris (1975) and Greer, Morris & Pettigale (1979). See also the work of Maguire and his associates (Maguire et. al., 1978, 1980). The report on the personal relationships of cancer survivors was by Leiber et. al. (1976). See Greer & Silberfarb (1982) for a good review of some of the work on both retrospective and contiguous studies.

The major prospective studies are described in the following works; The Johns Hopkins studies are summarized in five volumes by Thomas et. al. (in particular volumes 4 & 5, 1976, 1982. See also Thomas, Duszynski & Shaffer, 1979). The Swedish study was described by Hagnell (1966) and a review of the Berkeley study can be found in Holden (1978). The Yugoslav study's results have been published by Grossarth-Maticek and his associates (1983a, b, 1985). The Harvard and Pensylvania Universities study is still underway but some reports have been published; see for example Paffenberger et. al. (1977, 1978), Paffenberger, Kampert & Chang (1980) and Whittemore et. al. (1983, 1984). The Kansas study is described in Dattore, Shontz & Coyne (1980).

A useful review of studies on cancer and stress in animals is Riley et. al. (1981). See also Riley (1975) and Sklar & Anisman (1979, 1980).

Books and articles I have found useful on alternative medical approaches to cancer treatment are; Cade (1977), Cade & Coxhead (1979), Forbes (1984), Garner (1974), Griffin (1974), Issels (1970, 1971), Kinlen et. al. (1983), Kidman (1983) Magarey (1981, 1983), Meares, (1979, 1980), Moss (1980),

Simonton, Mathews-Simonton & Creighton (1980), Simonton (1983), Stefanson (1960) & Tropp (1980).

CHAPTER 3   A NEW PSYCHOLOGY OF CANCER

A number of authors have influenced my thinking about how to develop a new model for the psychology of cancer. I have always been intrigued by the possibilities inherent in General Systems Theory for psychosomatic medicine and the writings of Von Bertalanfy (1955, 1964, 1968) offer an excellent introduction to the biology and psychology based on it. His books also have the advantage of being quite readable.

More specifically though the following works on psychology, biology, psychiatry and psychosomatic medicine give some idea of current approaches to the relationships of stress, society and personality to illness: Ader (1980), Changeux (1984), Creed & Pfeffer (1982), Cox (1978), Dohrenwend & Dohrenwend (1974), Dubos, (1959, 1968) Fries (1980), Grenell & Gabay (1976), Hansell (1976), Hill (1976), Illich (1976), Kissen (1969), Lipowski (1977, 1984), Miller, Gallanter & Pribram (1960), Pribram (1962), Pribram (1970), Lowenthal & Haven (1968), Meerwein (1978), Meyersburg & Post (1979), Marmor (1983), Marmor & Woods (1980), Reed, McGee & Yano (1984), Schultz (1970), Schwartz & Weiss (1977), Sontag (1977), Syme (1974), Von Bonsdorf (1981), Weiner (1982), Weiss et. al. (1981), Wilf et. al. (1983).

However we define the effects of personality, stress or emotional upset in the individual we know that these effects are mediated by the body's central nervous, endocrine and immune systems. In trying to show how these systems are linked to cancer and to human behaviour I have drawn on the following articles; Besedovsky et. al. (1979), Bieliauskas & Garron (1982), Cunningham (1981), Fox (1981), Jemmott & Locke (1984), Leibowitz & Hughes (1983), Maclean & Reichlin (1981), Minter & Kimball (1978), Murray Parkes, Benjamin & Fitzgerald (1969), Rogers, Dubey & Reich (1979), Sklar & Anisman (1981), Visintainer, Seligman & Volpicelli (1983) & Stein (1983).

The papers on Natural Killer Cell Activity (NKCA) are by Locke et. al. (1984) and Heisel et. al. (1985). The Columbus, Ohio studies are described in Kiecolt-Glaser (1984a, b).

Much of the important work showing how the immune system may be conditioned by the CNS has been done by Ader and his associates; see in particular Ader (1983a, b), Ader, Cohen & Bovbjerg (1983) & Bovbjerg, Ader & Cohen (1982).

The important role played by relationships in the maturation and regulation of the three systems is well-demonstrated in the following works; Bartrop et. al. (1977), Butler, Suskind & Schanberg (1978), Cobb (1976), Hofer et. al. (1972), Hofer (1984), Schleifer et. al. (1983), & Vernikos-Danellis & Winget (1979). Related work on the importance of relationships for behaviour and other aspects of human function are; Argyle (1975), Davis (1971), Eibl-Eibesfeldt (1972), Morris (1982) & Scheflen (1972). Most of the latter are easy to read and offer insights into just how subtly human interaction shapes body activity.

CHAPTER 5 THE PSYCHOLOGY OF THE COMMON CANCERS

In preparing this chapter I found the following works of value, detailed according to area:

For lung cancer; Abse et. al. (1974), Blohmke, Von Engelhardt, & Stelzer (1984), Cornea et. al. (1983), Eysenck (1980), Grossarth-Maticek, et. al. (1983a, b, 1985), Grossarth-Maticek, Jancovic & Vetter (1982), Kissen (1963, 1967, 1969), Knoth, Bohn & Schmidt (1983), Lebovitz, Ostfeld & Moses (1972), Schmidt (1984), Thornton (1978), Wald et. al. (1980, 1983) & Wynder & Hecht (1976).

For cancers of the digestive tract; Burkitt (1971), Cotton (1981), Cummings (1978), Ellis (1983), Haenszel et. al. (1972), Harries, Baird & Rhodes (1982), Hirayama (1967), Holdstock et. al. (1984), Joossens & Geboers (1981, 1983), Ketikangas-Jarvinen & Loven (1983), Logan et. al. (1983, 1984), Lovett (1976), Macrae et. al. (1984), Merliss (1971), Mcdermott et. al. (1980), Riddell & Levin (1983), Sato et. al. (1959), Sherlock

(1982), Stubbs, (1983) & Whitehead & Bosmajian (1982).

For breast cancer; Anderson (1974), Baider & Sarell (1983), Barltrop & Kalache (1984), Bonadonna (1984), Becker (1979), Engelman & Craddick (1984), Faulder (1982), Fisher, Redmond & Fisher (1980), Gorzynski et. al. (1980), Helmrich et. al. (1983), Jansen & Muenz (1984), Klein (1971), Magarey, Todd & Blizard (1977), Marshall & Funch (1983), Masters & Johnson (1966), Morris et. al. (1980), Morris & Greer (1982), Paffenberger, Kampert & Chang (1980), Renneker (1963), Reznikoff (1955), Roberts (1984), Seely & Horrobun (1983), Todd & Magarey (1978), Waaler & Lund (1983), & Wirshing et. al. (1981, 1982).

For cancers of the genital regions; Asine, Shambaugh & Heise (1978), Cummings et. al. (1983), Garnick, Mayer & Richie (1980), Golden (1983), Hulka (1982), Kessler (1979, 1981), Lambert, Morisset & Bielmann (1980), Robinson (1985), Schottenfeld et. al. (1980) & Schottenfeld & Fraumeni (1982).

For skin cancers; Elwood et. al. (1984), Lee (1982), Lee & Strickland (1980), Mackie (1983), Mackie & Aitchison (1982) & Swerlow (1979).

I may have inadvertently given the impression by my lack of a case study of testicular cancer that this cancer, like penile cancer, is a rare condition. As I described earlier testicular cancer is relatively common. Unfortunately I have personally not had the kind of close contact with a case necessary to present it here.

CHAPTER 5　　PREVENTING CANCER

Precious little has been written about cancer prevention in general. Rosenbaum (1983) & Whelan (1980) are useful introductions to the area for the layperson.

I made use of the following works in preparing this chapter: Berkman & Syme (1979), Caplan (1974, 1981), Caplan & Killilea (1976), Coelho, Hamburg & Adams (1974), Frey (1984), Kaplan, Cassel & Gore (1977), Pearlin et. al. (1981), Revenson, Wollman & Felton (1983), Williams, Ware & Donald (1981) & Wortman & Lehman (1984).

CHAPTER 6   SURVIVING CANCER

The following general works were used in preparing this chapter;
Baider & Sarell (1984); Brunquell & Hall (1984), Craig &
Abeloff (1974), Eiser (1982), Falke & Taylor (1983), Foerster
(1984), Goldberg (1983), Gordon (1980), Holland (1981a, b),
Holland & Mastrovito (1980), Holland & Rowland (1981),
Honsalek (1983), Israel (1981), Langer, Janis & Wolfer (1975),
Lipowski (1983a, b), Louhivouri & Hakama (1979), Magni et.
al. (1983), Maguire (1983), Massie, Holland & Glass (1983),
Plumb & Holland (1977), Schmal et. al. (1983), Sellschop,
Ludeke & Haertal (1981), Silberfarb (1982), Silberfarb & Greer
(1982), Silberfarb, Maurer & Crouthamel (1980), Silberfarb,
Philibert & Levine (1980), Silberfarb & Levine (1980), Sobel &
Worden (1981), Wanlass & Prinz (1982), Wilson-Barnett
(1984), Wirsching & Wirsching (1980), Worden & Weisman
(1980) & Zimmermann, Drings & Wagner (1984).

Useful references dealing with how people cope with breast
cancer are as follows; Baider & Edelstein (1981), Bloom (1982),
Christensen et. al. (1982), Dean, Chetty & Forrest (1983),
Derogatis, Abeloff & Melisaratos (1979), Downing & Windsor
(1984), Ellisch, Jamison & Pasnau (1978), Engleman &
Craddick (1984), Funch & Marshall (1983, 1984), Funch &
Mettler (1982), Golden (1983), Hertoft (1983), Hughes (1982),
Jamison, Ellisch & Pasnau (1978), Maguire et. al. (1982),
Maguire (1980a, b), Messerli, Garamendi & Ramono (1980),
Morris, Greer & White (1977), Sachs et. al. (1981), Schwartz
(1977), Silberfarb (1978), Spiegel (1979), Spiegel et. al. (1981),
Spiegel & Bloom (1983a, b) & Wellisch, Jamison & Pasnau
(1978).

For cancers of the digestive tract the following references
are useful; Devlin, Plant & Griffen (1971), Keltikangas-
Jarvinen, Loven & Moller (1984), Kuchenhoff et. al. (1981),
Stodil (1983), Thomas, Madden & Jehu (1984) & Wirsching,
Drurier & Hermann (1975).

For cervical cancer; Moth (1983) & Bertelsen (1983) offer
useful advice.

On the effects of cancer treatments see; Allen (1978),
Altamier, Ross & Moore (1982), Berg (1983a, b), Bernstein

(1978), Burish & Lyles (1981), Cotanch (1983) Forester, Kornfeld & Fleiss (1978), Katz, Kellerman & Siegel (1980), Maguire et. al. (1980), Meadows & Evans (1976), Meyerowitz, Watkins & Sparks (1983), Nerenz, Leventhal & Love (1982), Nesser et. al. (1980), Palmer et. al. (1980), Peck & Boland (1977), Redd & Andrykowski (1982), Silberfarb (1983), Silberfarb et. al. (1983) & Weddington, Miller & Sweet (1984).

REFERENCES

Abse, D.W. et. al. (1974) Personality and behavioural characteristics of lung cancer patients. *Journal of Psychosomatic
Research*: 18, 101-13

Achte, K., & Pakaslahti, A. (Eds) (1981) Psychosomatic factors
in chronic illness. *Psychiatria Fennica Supplementum*
Proceedings of the symposium sponsored by the Gyllen-
berg Foundation, Espoo, Finland, December 1980

Ader, R. (1980) Psychosomatic and psychoimmunological
research. *Psychosomatic Medicine*, 42, 307-21

Ader, R. (Ed.) (1981) *Psychoneuroimmunology*. New York,
Academic Press

Ader, R. (1983a) Behavioural conditioning and immunity. N.
Fabris, E. Garaci, et. al. (Eds) *Immuno Regulation* New
York, Colin Plenum Publishing Corp.

Ader, R. (1983b) Developmental psychoneuroimmunology.
Developmental Psychology & Biology, 16, 251-67

Ader, R., Cohen, N., & Bovbjerg, D. (1983) Immuno-regulation
by behavioural conditioning. *Trends in Pharmacological
Sciences*, 4, 78-80

Alberts, B. et. al. (1983) *Molecular Biology of the Cell.* Garland

Allen, J.O. (1978) The effects of cancer therapy on the nervous
system *Journal of Pediatrics*, 93, 903-9

Altamier, E.M., Ross, W.E., & Moore, K. (1982) A pilot investigation of the psychological functioning of patients with anticipatory vomiting. *Cancer*, 49, 201-4

Ames, R.G. (1983) Gastric cancer and coal mine dust exposure. *Cancer*, 52, 1346-50

Anderson, D.E. (1974) Genetic study of breast cancer: Identification of a high risk group. *Cancer*, 34, 1090-7

Antonovsky, A. (1980) *Health, stress & coping* San Francisco: Jossey-Bass

Apfel, R.J. (1982) How are women sicker than men? *Psychotherapy and Psychosomatics*, 37, 106-18

Asine, A.J., Shambaugh, E.M., & Herse, H.W. (1978) Survival for individuals with cancers of the genital organs. *U.S. Dept of Health, Education & Welfare*, publ. 78-1543

Argyle, M. (1975) *Bodily Communication* London: Methuen

Bahnson, C.B. (1981) An historical family systems approach to coronary heart disease & cancer. In K.E. Schaeffer, et. al. (Eds) *A new image of man in medicine.* New York: Futura

Bahnson, C.B., & Bahnson, M.B. (1969) Ego defences in cancer patients. *Annals of the New York Academy of Science*, 164, 546-59

Baider, L. & Edelstein, E.L. (1981) Coping mechanisms of post mastectomy women. A group experience. *Israel Journal of Medical Sciences*, 17, 988-92

Baider, L., & Sarell, M. (1983) Perceptions and causal attributions of Israeli women with breast cancer concerning their illness, the effects of ethnicity and religiosity. *Psychotherapy & Psychosomatics*, 39, 136-43

Baider, L., & Sarell, M. (1984) Couples in crisis: patient-spouse differences in perception of interaction patterns and the illness situation. *Family Therapy*, 2, 115-112

Barker, D.J.P. (1984) Time trends in cancer mortality in England and Wales. *British Medical Journal*, 288, 1325-6

Barker, D.J.P., & Rose, G. (1976) *Epidemiology in Medical Practice.* London: Churchill Livingstone

Barltrop, K., & Kalache, A. (1984) Psychosocial aspects of breast cancer: an overview. Unpubl: Mss. University of Oxford.

Bartrop, R.W. (1979) The influence of the psyche and the brain on immunity and disease susceptibility. *Psychosomatic*

Medicine, 41, 147-64

Bartrop, R.W., et. al. (1977) Depressed lymphocyte function after bereavement. *Lancet*, 16 April, 834-6

Becker, H. (1979) Psychodynamic aspects of breast cancer. Differences in younger and older patients. *Psychotherapy & Psychosomatics*, 32, 287-96

Beresford, S.A.A. (1983) Cancer incidence and re-use of drinking water. *American Journal of Epidemiology*, 117, 258-68

Berg, R.A., et. al. (1983a) Neuropsychological sequelae of post-radiation somnolence syndrome *Developmental & Behavioural Paediatrics*, 4, 103-7

Berg, R.A., et. al. (1983b) The neuropsychological effects of acute lymphocytic leukaemia and its treatment — a 3-year report: intellectual functioning and academic achievement. *Clinical Neuropsychology*, 5, 9-13

Berkman, L.F., & Syme, S.L. (1979) Social networks, host resistance and mortality: a 9-year follow-up study of Alameda County residents. *American Journal of Epidemiology*, 109, 186-204

Bernstein, I.L. (1978) Taste aversions in children receiving chemotherapy. *Science*, 200, 1302-3

Bertelsen, K. (1983) Sexual dysfunction after treatment of cervical cancer. *Danish Medical Bulletin*, 50, 31-4

Besedovsky, H., et. al. (1979) Immunoregulation mediated by the sympathetic nervous system. *Cellular Immunology*, 48, 346-55

Berridge, M.J. (1985) The molecular basis of communication within the cell. *Scientific American*, 253, 124-35

Bieliauskas, L.A. & Garron, D.C. (1982) Psychological depression & cancer. *General Hospital Psychiatry*, 4, 187-95

Blohmke, M., Von Engelhardt, B., & Stelzer, O. (1984) Psychosocial factors and smoking as risk factors in lung carcinoma. *Journal of Psychosomatic Research*, 28, 221-9

Bloom, J.R. (1982) Social support, accommodation to stress and adjustment to breast cancer. *Social Science & Medicine*, 16, 91-8

Bloom, S. & Polak, J.M. (1981) *Gut hormones*. Edinburgh: Churchill Livingstone

Blot, W.J., et. al. (1983) Lung cancer among long-term steel workers. *American Journal of Epidemiology*, 177, 706-16

Bodley Scott, R. (1981) *Cancer.* Oxford: Oxford University Press

Bonadonna, G. (Ed.) (1984) *Breast cancer: diagnosis & management.* New York: Wiley

Bovbjerg, D., Ader, R., & Cohen, N. (1982) Behaviourally conditioned suppression of a graft-versus-host response. *Proceedings of the National Academy of Science*, 79, 583-5

Bovbjerg, D., Cohen, N., & Ader, R. (1982) The central nervous system & learning: a strategy for immune regulation. *Immunology Today*, 3, 287-91

Brunnquell, D., & Hall, M.D. (1984) Issues in the psychological care of pediatric oncology patients. In S. Chers & A. Thomas (Eds) *Annual progress in child psychiatry and child development* New York: Brunner/Mazel

Burish, T.G., & Lyles, J.N. (1981) Effectiveness of relaxation training in reducing adverse reactions to cancer chemotherapy. *Journal of Behavioural Medicine*, 4, 65-78

Burkitt, D.P. (1971) Epidemiology of cancer of the colon and rectum. *Cancer*, 28, 3

Burrows, J. (1983) *A Practical essay on cancer.* London

Butler, S.R., Suskind, M.R., & Schauberg, S. (1978) Maternal behaviour as a regulator of polyamic biosynthesis in brain and heart of the developing rat pup. *Science*, 199, 445-7

Cade, C.M. (1977) Biometric research into the healing process and the brain rhythms of healers. *Sixth annual conference of health and healing*: Wrekin Trust Lecture No. 69. Wrekin Trust, Little Birch, Hereford

Cade, C.M., & Coxhead, N. (1979) *The awakened mind.* New York, Declacorte

Caplan, G. (1974) *Support systems & community mental health.* New York: Behavioural Publications

Caplan, G. (1981) Mastery of stress: psychosocial aspects. *American Journal of Psychiatry*, 138, 413-20

Caplan, G., & Killilea, M. (Eds) (1976) *Support systems and mutual help.* New York: Grune & Stratton

Cassel, J. (1976) The contribution of the social environment to host resistance. *American Journal of Epidemiology*, 104, 107-23

Changeaux, J-P (1985) *Neuronal man: the biology of mind.* New

York: Pantheon

Christensen, K., et. al. (1982) Phantom breast syndrome in young women after mastectomy for breast cancer. *Acta. Chir. Scand.*, 148, 351-4

Cobb, S. (1976) Social support as a moderator of stress. *Psychosomatic Medicine*, 38, 300-14

Coelho, G.V., Hamburg, D.A., & Adams, J.E. (1974) *Coping and adaptation.* New York: Basic Books

Cotanch, P. (1983) Relaxation training for control of nausea and vomiting in patients receiving chemotherapy. *Cancer Nursing*, August, 277-83

Cooper, C.L. (1982) Psychosocial stress and cancer. *Bulletin of the British Psychological Society*, 35, 456-9

Cornea, R., et. al. (1983) Passive smoking and lung cancer. *Lancet*, ii, 595-7

Cotton, P.B. (Ed) (1981) *Early Gastric Cancer.* London: Smith, Kline & French

Cox, T (1978) *Stress.* London: Macmillan

Craig, T.J. & Abeloff, M.D. (1974) Psychiatric symptomotology among hospitalized cancer patients. *American Journal of Psychiatry*, 131, 1323-7

Creed, F., & Pfeffer, J.M. (Eds) (1982) *Medicine & psychiatry: a practical approach.* London: Pitman

Crisp, A.H. (1970) Some psychosomatic aspects of neoplasia. *British Journal of Medical Psychology*, 43, 313-31

Cummings, J.K. (1978) Dietary factors in the aetiology of gastrointestinal cancer. *Journal of Human Nutrition*, 32, 455-65

Cummings, K.M., et. al. (1983) What young men know about testicular cancer. *Preventive Medicine*, 12, 326-30

Cunningham, A.J. (1981) Mind, body and immune response. In Ader (1981)

Datton, P.J., Shontz, F.C., & Coyne, L. (1980) Premorbid personality differentiation of cancer and noncancer groups. *Journal of Consulting & Clinical Psychology*, 48, 388-94

Davis, F. (1971) *Inside Intuition.* New York: McGraw Hill

Dean, C., Chetty, U., & Forrest, A.P. (1983) Effects of immediate breast reconstruction on psychological morbidity after mastectomy. *Lancet*, 1, 459-62

Derogatis, L.R., Abeloff, M.D., & Melisaratos, N. (1979) Psychological coping mechanisms and survival time in metastatic breast cancer. *Journal of the American Medical Association*, 242, 1504-8

Devlin, B., Plant, J.A. & Griffen, M. (1971) Aftermath of surgery for anorectal cancer. *British Medical Journal*, 3, 413-8

Dohrenwend, E.S. & Dohrenwend, B.P. (1974) *Stressful life events: their nature and effects.* New York: John Wylie

Doll, R. (1972) Cancer in five continents. *Proceedings of the Royal Society of Medicine*, 65, 49

Doll, R., & Peto, R. (1981) *The cause of cancer.* Oxford: Oxford University Press

Downing, R., & Windsor, C.W.O. (1984) Disturbance of sensation after mastectomy. *British Medical Journal*, 1650, 2884

Dubos, R. (1959) *Mirage of health.* New York Harper & Row

Dubos, R. (1968) *Man, medicine & environment.* New York: The New American Library

Duff, R.S., & Hollingsheard, A.B. (1968) *Sickness & Society.* New York: Harper & Row

Eibl-Eibesfeldt, I. (1972) *Love & hate. The natural history of behaviour patterns.* New York: Holt, Rinehart & Winston

Eiser, J.R. (Ed) (1982) *Social psychology & behavioural medicine.* New York: Wiley

Ellis, H. (1983) Recurrent cancer of the large bowel. *British Medical Journal*, 287, 1741-2

Ellisch, D.K., Jamison, K.R., & Pasnau, R.O. (1978) Psychosocial aspects of mastectomy. 2. The man's perspective. *American Journal of Psychiatry*, 135, 543-6

Elwood, J.M., et. al. (1984) Pigmentation and skin reaction to sun as risk factors for cutaneous melanoma: Western Canada melanoma study. *British Medical Journal*, 288, 99-102.

Engel, G.L. (1977) The need for a new medical model: a challenge for biomedicine. *Science*, 196, 129-36

Engelman, S. & Craddick, R. (1984) The symbolic relationship of breast cancer patients to their cancer, cure, physician and themselves. *Psychotherapy & Psychosomatics*, 41, 68-76.

Eysenck, H.J. (1980) *The causes and effects of smoking.* London: Maurice Temple Smith

Fabris, N, & Garaci, E. et. al. (1983) *Immuno regulation.* New York: Plenum

Falke, R.L., & Taylor, S.E. (1983) Support groups for cancer patients. *UCLA Cancer Centre Bulletin,* Fall, 13-15

Faulder, C. (1982) *Breast Cancer.* London: Virago

Ferlic, M., Goldman, A., & Kennedy, B.J. (1979) Group counselling in adult patients with advanced cancer. *Cancer,* 43, 760-3

Fisher, B., Redmond, C., & Fisher, E.R. (1980) The contribution of recent NSABP clinical trials of primary breast cancer therapy to an understanding of tumor biology. An overview of findings. *Cancer,* 46, 1009

Foerster, K. (1984) Supportive psychotherapy combined with autogenous training in acute leukaemic patients under isolation therapy. *Psychotherapy & Psychosomatics,* 41, 100-5

Forester, B.M., Kornfeld, D.S., & Fleiss, J. (1978) Psychiatric aspects of radiotherapy. *American Journal of Psychiatry,* 135, 960-3

Forbes, A. (1984) *Cancer and its non-toxic treatment.* Bristol: Cancer Help Centre

Fox, B.H. (1981) Psychosocial factors and the immune system in human cancer. In Ader (1981)

Fraumeni, J.F. (Ed) (1975) *Persons at high risk of cancer.* New York: Academic Press

Frey, J. (1984) A family/systems approach to illness — maintaining behaviours in chronically ill adolescents. *Family Process,* 23, 251-60

Fries, J.F. (1980) Aging, natural death and the compression of morbidity. *New England Journal of Medicine,* July, 130-5

Funch, D.P., & Marshall, J. (1983) The role of stress, social effort and age in survival from breast cancer. *Journal of Psychosomatic Research,* 27, 77-84

Funch, D.P., & Marshall, J.R. (1984) Self reliance as a modifier of the effects of life stress and social support. *Journal of Psychosomatic Research,* 28, 9-16

Funch, D.P., & Mettler, C. (1982) The role of support in relation to recovery from breast cancer. *Social Science & Medicine*, 16, 91-8

Garner, J. (1974) Spontaneous regressions: scientific documentation as a basis for the declaration of miracles. *Canadian Medical Association Journal*, 111, 1254

Garnick, M.B., Mayer, R.J., & Richie, J.P. (1980) Testicular self-examination. *New England Journal of Medicine*, 302, 297

Gendron, D. (1701) *Enquiries into the nature, knowledge and cure of cancers.* London

Goldberg, R.J. (1983) Systematic understanding of cancer patients who refuse treatment. *Psychotherapy & Psychosomatics*, 39, 180-9

Goldberg, R., & Tull, R. (1983) *The psychosocial dimension of cancer.* New York: The Free Press

Golden, M. (1983) Female sexuality and crisis of mastectomy. *Danish Medical Bulletin*, 50, 13-16

Golden, J.S. (1983) Sex and cancer. *Danish Medical Bulletin*, 30, 4-6

Gordon, W.A., et. al. (1980) Efficacy of psychosocial intervention with cancer patients. *Journal of Consulting & Clinical Psychology*, 48, 743-59

Gorzynski, J.G., et. al. (1980) Stability of ego defences and endocrine responses in women prior to breast biopsy and 10 years later. *Psychosomatic Medicine*, 42, 323-8

Greer, S. & Morris, T. (1975) Psychological attributes of women who develop breast cancer: a controlled study. *Journal of Psychosomatic Research*, 19, 147-53

Greer, S., Morris, T., & Pettingale, K.W. (1979) Psychological response to breast cancer: effect on outcome. *Lancet*, 13th October, 785-7

Greer, S., & Silberfarb, P.M. (1982) Psychological concomitants of cancer: current state of research. *Psychological Medicine*, 12, 563-73

Gregory, R.A. (1982) Regulatory peptides of gut and brain. *British Medical Bulletin*, 38, 219-313

Grenell, R.G., & Gabay, S. (1976) *Biological foundations of psychiatry.* New York: Raven

Griffin, G.E. (1974) *World without cancer.* Westlake: American Media

Grossarth-Maticek, R., Jancovic, M., & Vetter, H. (1982) Standard risk factors for lung cancer, cardiac infarct, apoplexy, diabetes mellitus and the changes in psycho-social context. *Psychotherapy & Psychosomatics,* 37, 13-21

Grossarth-Maticek, R., et. al. (1983a) Smoking as a risk factor for lung cancer and cardiac infarct as mediated by psycho-social variables. A prospective investigation. *Psycho-therapy & Psychosomatics,* 39, 94-105

Grossarth-Maticek, R., et. al. (1983b) Psychosomatic factors involved in the process of cancerogenesis. Preliminary results of the Yugoslav prospective study. *Psychotherapy & Psychosomatics,* 40, 191-210

Grossarth-Maticek, R., Bastiaans, J., & Kanazir, D.T. (1985) Psychosocial factors as strong predictors of mortality from cancer, ischaemic heart disease and stroke: the Yugoslav prospective study. *Journal of Psychosomatic Research,* 29, 167-76

Haenszel, W., et. al. (1972) Stomach cancer among Japanese in Hawaii. *Journal of the National Cancer Institute,* 49, 969-88

Hagnell, O. (1966) The premorbid personality of persons who developed cancer in a total population investigated in 1947 and 1957. *Annals of the New York Academy of Science,* 125, 846-55

Hansell, N. (1976) *The person-in-distress: on the biologic dynamics of adaptation.* New York: Behavioral Publications

Harnden, D.G. (1983) Familial susceptibility to cancer. *British Medical Journal,* 286, 1531-2

Harries, A.D., Baird, A., & Rhodes, J. (1982) Non-smoking: a feature of ulcerative colitis. *British Medical Journal,* 284, 706

Heisel, J.S. et. al. (1985) Correlation of MMPI scores and Natural Killer Cell Activity in healthy college students. Unpublished Mss. Used with permission.

Helmrich, S.P., et. al. (1983) Risk factors for breast cancer. *American Journal of Epidemiology,* 117, 35-45

Hertoft, P. (1983) To be unreserved. *Danish Medical Bulletin,* 50, 30, 2-3

Hill, G.B. et. al. (1983) Trends in the incidence of cancer of the female breast and reproductive tract in Alberta, 1953-1977. *Preventive Medicine,* 12, 296-303

Hill, O.W. (Ed.) (1976) *Modern trends in psychosomatic medicine.* London: Butterworth

Hirayama, T. (1967) The epidemiology of cancer of the stomach in Japan with special reference to the role of diet. In R.J.C. Harris (Ed.) *Proceedings of the Ninth International Cancer Congress* Berlin: Springer-Verlag

Hofer, M.A., et. al. (1972) A psychoendocrine study of bereavement. *Psychosomatic Medicine,* 34, 481-507

Hofer, M.A. (1984) Relationships as regulators: a psychobiologic perspective on bereavement. *Psychosomatic Medicine,* 46, 183-97

Holden, C. (1978) Cancer and the mind. How are they connected? *Science,* 200, 1363-9

Holdstock, G., et. al. (1984) Should patients with inflammatory bowel disease smoke? *British Medical Journal,* 288, 362

Holland, J.F. (1981a) Patients who seek unproven cancer remedies: a psychological perspective. *Clinical Bulletin,* 11, 102-5

Holland, J.C. (1981b) Stress and coping: families and terminal illness. *Stress & Coping,* Philadelphia Smith, Klein & French Laboratories, Report No. 2

Holland, J.C., & Frei, E. (1978) *Cancer Medicine.* Philadelphia: Lea & Febiger

Holland, J.C., & Mastrovito, R. (1980) Psychologic adaptation to breast cancer. *Cancer,* 46, 1045-52

Holland, J.C., & Rowland, J.H. (1981) Psychiatric, psychosocial and behavioural interventions in the treatment of cancer. In Weiss et. al.

Honsalek, I. (1983) Das Behandlungsteam des Karzinom — und des Leukaemiepatienten. *Schweiz. Rundschau Med,* 72, 44-8

Hughes, J. (1982) Emotional reactions to the diagnosis and treatment of early breast cancer. *Journal of Psychosomatic Research,* 26, 277-83

Hulka, B.S. (1982) Risk factors for cervical cancer. *Journal of Chronic Disease,* 35, 3-11

Illich, I. (1976) *Medical Nemesis: the expropriation of health.* London: Penguin.

Israel, L. (1981) *Conquering cancer.* Harmondsworth: Penguin

Issels, J. (1970) Immunotherapy in progressive metastatic cancer. *Clinical Trials Journal,* 7, 357-66

Issels, J. (1971) On a report about the treatment of cancer at the Ringberg-Klinik. *Krebsgeschehen,* 3, 54-104

Jacobs, T.J., & Charles, E. (1980) Life events in the occurrence of cancer in children. *Psychosomatic Medicine,* 42, 11-24

Jamison, K.R., Ellisch, D.K., & Pasnau, R.O. (1978) Psycho-social aspects of mastectomy. 1. The woman's perspective. *American Journal of Psychiatry,* 135, 432-6

Jansen, M.A., & Muenz, L.R. (1984) A retrospective study of personality variables associated with fibrocystic disease and breast cancer. *Journal of Psychosomatic Research,* 28, 35-42

Jemmott, J.B., & Locke, S.E. (1984) Psychosocial factors, immunologic mediation and human susceptibility to infectious diseases: how much do we know? *Psychological Bulletin,* 95, 78-108

Joossens, J.V., & Geboers, J. (1981) Nutrition and gastric cancer. *Nutrition and Cancer,* 2, 250-61

Joossens, J.V., & Geboers, J. (1983) Diet and environment in the etiology of gastric cancer. In R. Riddell & B. Levin (Eds) *Frontiers of gastrointestinal cancer.* New York: Elsevier

Kaplan, B., Cassel, J., & Gore, S. (1977) Social support and health. *Medical Care,* 15, 47-58

Katz, E.R., Kellerman, J., & Siegel, S.E. (1980) Behavioural distress in children with cancer undergoing medical procedures: developmental considerations. *Journal of Consulting & Clinical Psychology,* 48, 356-65

Katzenellenbogen, B. (1980) Dynamics of steroid hormone receptor action. *Annual Review of Physiology,* 42, 17-35

Keller, A.Z. (1983) Selected factors in the risks of upper alimentary cancers. *Preventive Medicine,* 12, 541-53

Kelley, P.T. (1983) Families and cancer: the role of inheritance. *Can you prevent cancer?* St. Louis: C.V. Mosby

Kessler, I.I. (1979) On the etiology & prevention of cervical cancer — a status report *Obstetrics & Gynaecology Survey*, 34, 790-4

Kessler, I.I. (1981) Etiological concepts in cervical carcinogenesis. *Gynaecological Oncology*, 12, 57-524

Keltikangas-Jarvinen, L., & Loven, E. (1983) Stability of personality dimensions related to cancer and colitis ulcerosa: a preliminary report. *Psychological Reports*, 52, 961-2.

Keltikangas-Jarvinen, L., Loven, E., & Moller, C. (1984) Psychic factors determining the long-term adaptation of colostomy and ileostomy patients. *Psychotherapy & Psychosomatics*, 41, 153-9

Knoth, A., Bohn, H., & Schmidt, F. (1983) Passivrauchen als Lungen Krebssursache bei Nichtraucherinnen. *Med. Kiln. Praxis*, 78, 54-9

Kidman, B. (1983) *A gentle way with cancer*. London: Century

Kiecolt-Glaser, J., et. al. (1984a) Psychosocial modifiers of immunocompetence in medical students. *Psychosomatic Medicine*, 46, 7-14

Kiecolt-Glaser, J., et. al. (1984b) Urinary cortisol levels, cellular immunocompetency and loneliness in psychiatric in-patients. *Psychosomatic Medicine*, 46, 15-23

Kinlen, L.J., Hennon, C., & Smith, P.G. (1983) A proportionate study of cancer mortality among members of a vegetarian society. *British Journal of Cancer*, 48, 355-61

Kissen, D.M. (1963) Personality characteristics in males conducive to lung cancer. *British Journal of Medical Psychology*, 35, 27-36

Kissen, D.M. (1967) The significance of personality in lung cancer in men aged 55-64. *British Journal of Medical Psychology*, 40, 29-43

Kissen, D.M. (1969) The present status of psychosomatic cancer research. *Geriatrics*, 24, 1929

Klauber, M.R., & Lyon, J.L. (1978) Gastric cancer in a coal mining region. *Cancer*, 41, 2355-8

Klein, R. (1971) A crisis to grow on. *Cancer*, 28, 1660-5

Kowal, S.J. (1955) Emotions as a cause of cancer: 18th and 19th century contributions. *Psychoanalytic Review*, 42, 217-27

Krasnoff, A. (1959) Psychological variables in human cancer.

Psychosomatic Medicine, 21, 291-5

Krieger, D.T. (1983) Brain peptides: what, where and why. *Science*, 222, 975-85

Kuchenhoff, J. et. al. (1981) Coping with a stoma — a comparative study of patients with rectal carcinoma or inflammatory bowel diseases. *Psychotherapy and Psychosomatics*, 36, 98-104

Lambert, B., Morisset, R., & Bielmann, P. (1980) An etiologic survey of clinical factors in cervical intraepithelial neoplasia. *Journal of Reproductive Medicine*, 24, 26-31

Land, H., Parada, L.F., & Weniberg, R.A. (1983) Tumorigenic conversion of primary embryo fibroblasts requires at least two co-operating oncogenes. *Nature*, 304, 596-602

Langer, E.J., Jamis, I.L., & Wolfer, J.A. (1975) Reduction of psychological stress in surgical patients. *Journal of Experimental Social Psychology*, 11, 155-65

Lebovits, B., Ostfeld, A.M., & Moses, V.K. (1972) Cigarette smoking and personality. *Journal of Chronic Diseases*, 25, 581

Lee, J.A.H. (1982) Melanoma and exposure to sunlight. *Epidemiology Review*, 4, 110-36

Lee, J.A.H., & Strickland, D. (1980) Malignant melanoma: social status and outdoor work. *British Journal of Cancer*, 41, 757-63

Leiber, L., et. al. (1976) Communication of affection between cancer patients and their spouses. *Psychosomatic Medicine*, 38, 379-89

Leibowitz, S., & Hughes, R.A.C. (1983) *Immunology of the nervous system.* London: Edward Arnold

Lermer, S. (1982) *Cancer and the psyche: medicine in self-help.* Munich: Causa

Levine, P.M., Silberfarb, P.M., & Lipowski, Z.J. (1978) Mental disorders in cancer patients: a study of 100 psychiatric referrals. *Cancer*, 42, 1385-91

Le Shan, L. (1959) Psychological states as factors in the development of malignant disease: a critical review. *Journal of the National Cancer Institute*, 22, 1-18

Le Shan, L. (1966) An emotional life history pattern associated with neoplastic disease. *Annals of New York Academy of*

Science, 125, 780-93

Le Shan, S. (1984) *You can fight for your life.* Wellingborough: Thorsons

Liddell, F.D.K. (1973) Mortality of British coal miners in 1961. *British Journal of Industrial Medicine*, 30, 15-24

Lipowski, Z.J. (1977) Psychosomatic medicine in the seventies: an overview. *American Journal of Psychiatry*, 134, 233-44

Lipowski, Z.J. (1983a) The need to integrate liaison psychiatry and geropsychiatry. *American Journal of Psychiatry*, 140, 1003-5

Lipowski, Z.J. (1983b) Current trends in consultation-liaison psychiatry. *Canadian Journal of Psychiatry*, 28, 329-38

Lipowski, Z.J. (1984) What does the word 'psychosomatic' really mean? *Psychosomatic Medicine*, 46, 153-71

Lips, K.J.M. et. al. (1982) Genetic predisposition to cancer in man. *American Journal of Medicine*, 73, 305-7

Locke, S.E. (1983) Stress, personality and cancer. In E.H. Rosenbaum (Ed.) *Can you prevent cancer?* St Louis: C.V. Mosby

Locke, S., et. al. (1984) Life change stress, psychiatric symptoms and Natural Killer Cell Activity. *Psychosomatic Medicine*, 46

Logan, J., & Cairns, J. (1982) The secrets of cancer. *Nature*, 300, 104-5

Logan, R.F.A., et. al. (1983) Is cigarette smoking associated with Crohn's Disease? *Gut*, 24, A980

Logan, R.F.A., et. al. (1984) Smoking and ulcerative colitis. *British Medical Journal*, 288, 751-3

Louhivuori, K.A., & Hakama, M. (1979) Risk of suicide among cancer patients. *American Journal of Epidemiology*, 109, 59-65

Lovett, E. (1976) Family studies in cancer of the colon and rectum. *British Journal of Surgery*, 63, 13-8

Lowenthal, M.F., & Hanen, C. (1968) Interaction and adaptation; intimacy as a critical variable. *American Sociological Review*, 33, 20-30

Macek, C. (1982) Of mind and mobility: can stress and grief depress immunity. *Journal of the American Medical Association*, 248, 405-7

Mackie, R.M. (1983) The pathogenesis of cutaneous malignant melanoma. *British Medical Journal*, 287, 1568-9

Mackie, R.M., & Aitchison, T.C. (1982) Severe sunburn and subsequent risk of primary cutaneous malignant melanoma in Scotland. *British Journal of Cancer*, 46, 955-60

Maclean, D., & Reichlin, S. (1981) Neuroendocrinology and the immune response. In Ader (1981)

Macrae, F.A., et. al. (1984) Predicting colon cancer screening behaviour from health beliefs. *Preventive Medicine*, 13, 115-26

Magarey, C. (1981) Healing and meditation in medical practice. *Medical Journal of Australia*, 1, 338-41

Magarey, C. (1983) Holistic cancer therapy. *Journal of Psychosomatic Research*, 27, 181-4

Magarey, C.J., Todd, P.B., & Blizard, P.J. (1977) Psycho-social factors influencing delay and breast examination in women with symptoms of breast cancer. *Social Science & Medicine*, 11, 229-32

Magni, G., Messina, C., et. al. (1983) Psychological distress in parents of children with acute lymphatic leukaemia. *Acta Psychiatr. Scand*, 68, 297-300

Maguire, P. (1980) The repercussions of mastectomy on the family. *International Journal of Family Psychiatry*, 1, 485-503

Maguire, P. (1983) Psychiatric problems of mutilating surgery. *Medicine*, 1576-9

Maguire, G.P., et. al. (1978) Psychiatric problems in the first year after mastectomy. *British Medical Journal*, 1, 963-5

Maguire, P., et. al. (1980a) Psychiatric morbidity and the physical toxicity associated with adjuvant chemotherapy after mastectomy. *British Medical Journal*, 281, 1179-80

Maguire, P., et. al. (1980b) Effective counselling of the psychiatric mobility associated with mastectomy. *British Medical Journal*, 281, 1454-6

Maguire, P., et. al. (1982) Cost of counselling women who undergo mastectomy. *British Medical Journal*, 284, 1933-5

Marmor, J. (1983) Systems thinking in psychiatry: some theoretical and clinical implications. *American Journal of Psychiatry*, 140, 833-8

Marmor, J., & Woods, S.M. (1980) *The interface between the psychoanalytic and behaviour therapies.* New York: Plenum

Marshall, J.R., & Funch, D.P. (1983) Social environment and breast cancer. *Cancer,* 52, 1546-50

Mason, A.S. (1976) *Hormones and the body.* Revised Ed. Harmondsworth: Penguin

Massie, M.J., Holland, J., & Glass, E. (1983) Delirium in terminally ill cancer patients. *American Journal of Psychiatry,* 140, 1048-50

Masters, W.H., & Johnson, V.E. (1966) *Human sexual response.* Boston: Little Brown

McDermott, F.T., et. al. (1980) Changing survival prospects in carcinoma of the rectum. *British Journal of Surgery,* 67, 775-80

McIntyre, O.R. (1979) Current concepts in cancer: multiple myeloma. *New England Journal of Medicine,* 301, 193-6

McKegney, F.P. (1979) Mind & cancer. *Lancet,* 31 March, 706-7

Meadows, A.T., & Evans, A.E. (1976) Effects of chemotherapy on the central nervous system. *Cancer,* 37, 1079-85

Meares, A. (1979) Atavistic communication by touch in psychological treatment of cancer by intensive meditation. *Journal of Holistic Health,* 4, 120

Meares, A. (1980) What can a cancer patient expect from intensive meditation. *Australian Family Physician,* 9, 322

Meerwein, F. (1978) La psychologie du cancereux. *Folia Psychopractica,* Bâle: Hoffman-La Roche

Merliss, R.R. (1971) Talc, treated rice and Japanese stomach cancer. *Science,* 173, 1141-2

Messerli, M.C., Garamendi, C., & Ramono, J. (1980) Breast cancer: information as a technique of crisis intervention. *American Journal of Orthopsychiatry,* 50, 728-31

Meyerowitz, B., Watkins, I.K., & Sparks, F.C. (1983) Psychosocial implications of adjuvant chemotherapy. *Cancer,* 52, 1541-5

Meyersburg, H.A., & Post, R.M. (1979) An holistic developmental view of neural and psychological processes: a neurobiologic-psychoanalytic integration. *British Journal of*

Psychiatry, 135, 139-55

Miller, G.A., Gallanter, E., & Pribram, K.R. (1960) *Plans and the structure of behaviour.* New York: Holt

Miller, L.H., Ross, R., & Cohen, S.I. (1982) Stress: what can be done? *Bostonian Magazine*: 56, 13

Miller, T., & Spratt, J.S. (1979) Critical review of reported psychological correlates of cancer prognosis and growth. In Stoll (1979)

Minter, R.E., & Kimball, C.R. (1978) Life events and illness onset: a review. *Psychosomatics*, 19, 334-9

Morehead, R.R. (1965) *Human Patholoy.* New York: McGraw Hill

Morris, D. (1982) *Manwatching.* London: Triad

Morris, T., Greer, S., & White, P. (1977) Psychological and social adjustment to mastectomy: a two-year follow-up study. *Cancer*, 40, 2381-7

Morris, T., Greer, S., et. al. (1981) Patterns of expression of anger and their psychological correlates in women with breast cancer. *Journal of Psychosomatic Research*, 25, 111-7

Morris, T., & Greer, S. (1982) Psychological characteristics of women electing to attend a breast screening clinic. *Clinical Oncology*, 8, 113-9

Moss, G.E. (1973) *Illness, immunity and social interaction.* New York: Wylie

Moss, R.W. (1980) *The cancer syndrome.* New York: Grove Press

Moth, I., et. al. (1983) Sexual function and somatophysic reactions after vulvectomy. *Danish Medical Bulletin*, 30, 27-30

Murray, J.B. (1980) Psychosomatic aspects of cancer: an overview. *Journal of Genetic Psychology*, 136, 185-94

Murray Parkes, C., Benjamin, B., & Fitzgerald, R.G. (1969) Broken heart: a statistical study of increased mortality amongst widows. *British Medical Journal*, 1, 740-3

Najem, G.R., & Molteni, K.H. (1983) Respiratory organ cancer mortality in New Jersey counties and their relationship with selected demographic and environmental variables. *Preventive Medicine*, 12, 479-90

Nerenz, D.R., Leventhal, H., & Love, R. (1982) Factors contributing to emotional distress during cancer chemotherapy. *Cancer*, 50, 1020-7

Nesser, E.M., et. al. (1980) Pre-treatment nausea in cancer chemotherapy: a conditioned response? *Psychosomatic Medicine*, 42, 33-6

Novack, D.H., et. al. (1979) Changes in physicians' attitudes toward telling the cancer patient. *Journal of the American Medical Association*, 241, 897-900

Oken, D. (1961) What to tell cancer patients: a study of medical attitudes. *Journal of the American Medical Association*, 175, 1120-8

Osmond, C., et. al. (1983) *Trends in cancer mortality analysis by period of birth and death*. London: HMSO

Paffenberger, R.S., Wing, A.L., & Hyde, R.T. (1977) Characteristics in youth indicative of adult-onset Hodgkins Disease. *Journal of the National Cancer Institute*, 58, 1489-91

Paffenberger, R.S., Wing, A.L., & Hyde, R.T. (1978) Characteristics in youth predictive of adult-onset malignant lymphomas, melanomas and leukaemias. *Journal of the National Cancer Institute*, 60, 89-92

Paffenberger, R.S., Kampert, J.B., & Chang, H.G. (1980) Characteristics that predict risk of breast cancer before and after the menopause. *American Journal of Epidemiology*, 112, 258-68

Palmer, B.V., et. al. (1980) Adjuvant chemotherapy for breast cancer: side-effects and quality of life. *British Medical Journal*, 281, 1594-7

Palmer, G., & Scott, W.D. (1981) Lung cancer in ferrous foundry workers: a review. *American Industrial Hygiene Association Journal*, 42: 329-40

Pearlin, L., et. al. (1981) The stress process. *Journal of Health and Social Behaviour*, 22, 337-56

Peck, A., & Boland, J. (1977) Emotional reactions to radiation treatment. *Cancer*, 40, 180-4

Polak, J.M., & Bloom, S.R. (1983) Regulatory peptides: key factors in the control of bodily functions. *British Medical Journal*, 286, 1461-6

Polak, J.M., & Van Noorden, S. (1983) *Immunocytochemistry*

— *practical applications in pathology and biology.* Bristol: John Wright

Polakoff, P., & Rosenbaum, E.H. (1983) Environmental and occupational risks. In E.H. Rosenbaum (Ed.) *Can you prevent cancer?* St Louis: C.V. Mosby

Plumb, M.M., & Holland, J. (1977) Comparative studies of psychological function in patients with advanced cancer. 1. Self-reported depressive symptoms. *Psychosomatic Medicine,* 39, 264-76

Pribram, K.H. (1962) Interrelations of psychology and the neurological disciplines. In S. Koch (Ed) *Psychology: the study of a science. Volume 4.* New York: McGraw Hill.

Pribram, K.R. (1979) On knowing. Stanford University Department of Neurology

Rabkin, J.G., & Struening, E.L. (1976) Life events, stress and illness. *Science,* 194, 1013

Rather, L.J. (1978) *The genesis of cancer.* Baltimore: Johns Hopkins

Redd, W.H., & Andrykowski, M.A. (1982) Behavioural intervention in cancer treatment: controlling aversion reactions to chemotherapy. *Journal of Consulting and Clinical Psychology,* 50, 1018-29

Reed, D., McGee, D., & Yano, K. (1984) Psychosocial processes and the general susceptibility to chronic disease. *American Journal of Epidemiology,* 119, 356-70

Reif, A.E. (1983) Susceptibility to cancer and spontaneous incidence. *Oncology,* 40, 210-70

Renneker, R., et. al. (1963) Psychoanalytic explorations of emotional correlates of cancer of the breast. *Psychosomatic Medicine,* 25, No 2

Revenson, T.A., Wollman, C.A., & Felton, B. (1983) Social supports as stress buffers for adult cancer patients. *Psychosomatic Medicine,* 45, 321-31

Reznikoff, M. (1955) Psychological factors in breast cancer. *Psychosomatic Medicine,* 27, No 2

Riddell, R., & Levin, B. (Eds) (1983) *Frontiers of gastrointestinal cancer.* New York: Elseview

Riley, V. (1975) Mouse mammary tumors: alteration of incidence as apparent function of stress. *Science,* 189, 465-7

Riley, V., et. al. (1981) Psychoneuroimmunologic factors in neoplasia: studies in animals. In Ader (1981)

Roberts, M.M. (1984) Risk of breast cancer in women with history of benign disease of the breast. *British Medical Journal*, 288, 275-8

Robertson, M. (1983) Oncogenes and the origins of human cancer. *British Medical Journal*, 286, 81-2(a)

Robertson, M. (1983) Oncogenes and multistep carcinogenesis. *British Medical Journal*, 287, 1084-8(b)

Robinson, J. (1985) Not just casual sex. *The Observer*, 31 March, 49

Rogers, M.P., Duhey, D., & Reich, P. (1979) The influence of the psyche and the brain on immunity and susceptibility: a critical review. *Psychosomatic Medicine*, 41, 147-64

Rosenbaum, E.H. (Ed.) (1983) *Can you prevent cancer?* St Louis: C.V. Mosby

Rubens, R.D., & Knight, R.K. (1980) *Clinical oncology.* London: Hodder & Stoughton

Sachs, S., et. al. (1981) Comparative results of post-mastectomy rehabilitation in a specialized and community hospital. *Cancer*, 48, 1251-5

Sanger, C.K., & Rezinkoff, M. (1981) A comparison of the psychological effects of breast-saving procedures with the modified radical mastectomy. *Cancer*, 48, 2341-6

Sato, T., et. al. (1959) Studies of the causation of gastric cancer. *Bulletin of the Institute of Public Health*, 8, 187-98

Scheflen, A. (1972) *Body language and the social order.* Englewood Cliffe: Prentice Hall

Schmal, A.H., et. al. (1983) Well being of cancer survivors. *Psychosomatic Medicine*, 45, 163-9

Schmidt, F. (1984) Passive smoking and lung cancer. *Lancet*, 684

Schottenfeld, D., et. el. (1980) The epidemiology of testicular cancer in young adults. *American Journal of Epidemiology*, 112, 232-46

Schottenfeld, D., & Fraumeni, J.F. (Eds) (1982) *Cancer epidemiology and prevention.* Philadelphia: Saunders

Schleifer, S.J., et. al. (1983) Suppression of lymphocyte stimulation following bereavement. *Journal of the American*

Medical Association, 250, 374-7

Schmale, A., & Iker, H. (1966) The effects of hopelessness and the development of cancer. *Psychosomatic Medicine,* 28, 714-21

Schultz, D.P. (Ed.) (1970) *The science of psychology: critical reflections.* New York: Appleton-Century-Crofts

Schwartz, G.E., & Weiss, S.M. (1977) What is behavioural medicine? *Psychosomatic Medicine,* 377-81

Schwartz, M.D. (1979) An information and discussion programme for women after mastectomy. *Archives of Surgery,* 112, 276-81

Seely, S., & Horrobin, D.F. (1983) Diet and breast cancer: the possible connection with sugar consumption. *Medical Hypotheses,* 11, 319-27

Sellschopp, A., Ludeke, H., & Haertel, G. (1981) Structure and functions of the Heidelberg University Organization for after-care of cancer patients. *Psychotherapy & Psychosomatics,* 36, 17-23

Sherlock, P. (Ed.) (1982) *Precancerous conditions of the gastric intestinal tract.* New York: Raven

Silberfarb, P.M. (1978) Psychiatric themes in the rehabilitation of mastectomy patients. *International Journal of Psychiatry in Medicine,* 8, 159-67

Silberfarb, P.M. (1982) Research in adaptation to illness and psychosocial intervention. *Cancer,* 50, 1921-7

Silberfarb, P.M. (1983) Chemotherapy and cognitive defects in cancer patients. *Annual Review of Medicine,* 34, 35-46

Silberfarb, P.M., et. al. (1983) Psychological response of patients receiving two drug regimens for lung carcinoma. *American Journal of Psychotherapy,* 140, 110-1

Silberfarb, P.M., & Greer, S. (1982) Psychological concomitants of cancer: clinical aspect. *American Journal of Psychotherapy,* 36, 470-8

Silberfarb, P.M., & Levine, P.M. (1980) Psychosocial aspects of neoplastic disease. 3. Group support for the oncology nurse. *General Hospital Psychiatry,* 3, 192-7

Silberfarb, P.M., Maurer, L.H., & Crouthamel, C.S. (1980) Psychosocial aspects of neoplastic disease. 1. Functional status of breast cancer patients during different treatment regimens. *American Journal of Psychiatry*, 137, 450-5

Silberfarb, P.M., Philibert, D., & Levine, P.M. (1980) Psycho-social aspects of neoplastic disease. 2. Effective and cognitive effects of chemotherapy in cancer patients. *American Journal of Psychiatry*, 137, 597-601

Simonton, O.C., Mathews-Simonton, S., & Creighton, J.L. (1980) *Getting well again.* New York: Bantam

Simonton, O.C. (1983) Interview. *Journal of Alternative Medicine*, August, p. 2

Sklar, L.S., & Anisman, H. (1979) Stress and coping factors influence tumor growth. *Science*, 205, 513-5

Sklar, L.S., & Anisman, H. (1980) Social stress influences tumor growth. *Psychosomatic Medicine*, 42, 347-65

Sklar, L.S., & Anisman, H. (1981) Stress and cancer. *Psychological Bulletin*, 89, 369-406

Snyder, S.H. (1984) Drug and neurotransmitter receptors in the brain. *Science*, 224, 22-31

Snyder, S.H. (1985) The molecular basis of communication between cells. *Scientific American*, 253, 114-23

Sobel, H.J., & Worden, J.W. (1981) *Helping cancer patients cope.* New York: Guilford

Sontag, S. (1977) *Illness as metaphor.* New York: Farrar, Straus & Giroux

Spiegel, D. (1979) Psychological support for women with meta-static carcinoma. *Psychosomatics*, 20, 780-7

Spiegel, D., & Bloom, J.R. (1983a) Pain in metastatic breast cancer. *Cancer*, 52, 341-5

Spiegel, D., & Bloom, J.R. (1983b) Group therapy and hypnosis reduce metastatic breast carcinoma pain. *Psychosomatic Medicine*, 45, 333-9

Spiegel, D., Bloom, J.R., & Yalom, I. (1981) Group support for patients with metastatic cancer. *Archives of General Psychiatry*, 38, 527-33

Stodil, F. (1983) Intestinal stomas. *Danish Medical Bulletin*, 50, 35-7

Stefanson, V. (1960) *Cancer: disease of civilization?* New York: Hill & Wang

Steinhagen, A., et. al. (1983) Occupational risk factors in liver cancer: a retrospective case control study of primary liver cancer in New Jersey. *American Journal of Epidemiology*, 117, 443-54

Stein, M. (1981) A biophysical approach to immune function and medical disorders. *Pediatric Clinics of North America*, 4, 203-21

Stocks, P., & Davies, R.I. (1960) Epidemiological evidence from chemical and spectographic analyses that soil is concerned in the causation of cancer. *British Journal of Cancer*, 14, 8

Stoll, B.A. (1979) *Mind and cancer prognosis.* New York: Wiley

Stubbs, R.S. (1983) The aetiology of colorectal cancer. *British Journal of Surgery*, 70, 313-6

Swerdlow, A.J. (1979) Incidence of malignant melonoma of the skin in England and Wales and its relationship to sunshine. *British Medical Journal*, 1324-7

Swerdlow, A.J. (1983) Epidemiology of eye cancer in England and Wales, 1962-1977. *American Journal of Epidemiology*, 118, 294-300

Syme, S. (1974) Behavioural factors associated with the etiology of physical disease: a social epidemiological approach. *American Journal of Public Health*, 64, 1043-5

Tabin, C.J., et. al. (1982) Mechanism of activation of a human oncogene. *Nature*, 300, 143-9

Taylor, P. (1984) *The smoke ring.* New York: Pantheon

Thomas, C., Madden, F., & Jehu, D. (1984) Psychosocial morbidity in the first three months following stoma surgery. *Journal of Psychosomatic Research*, 28, 251-7

Thomas, C.B., et. al. (1976) *The precursors study: collected papers: volume 4.* Baltimore: The Johns Hopkins University School of Medicine

Thomas, C.B., et. al. (1982) *The precursors study: collected papers: volume 5* Baltimore: The Johns Hopkins University School of Medicine

Thomas, C.B., Duszynski, K.R., & Shaffer, J.W. (1979) Family attitudes reported in youth as potential predictors of cancer. *Psychosomatic Medicine*, 41, 287-302

Thornton, R.E. (Ed.) (1978) *Smoking behaviour: physiological and psychological influences.* Edinburgh: Churchill Livingstone

Todd, P.B., & Magarey, C.J. (1978) Ego defences and effects in women with breast symptoms: a preliminary measurement paradigm. *British Journal of Medical Psychology*, 51, 177-89

Tonegawa, S. (1985) The molecules of the immune system. *Scientific American*, 253, 104-13

Totman, R. (1979) *Social causes of illness*. London: Souvenn

Trillin, A.S. (1981) Of dragons and garden peas. A cancer patient talks to doctors. *New England Journal of Medicine*, 304, 699-701

Tropp, J. (1980) *Cancer, a healing crisis*. New York: Exposition Press

Vernikos-Danellis, J., & Winget, C.M. (1979) The importance of light, postural and social cues in the regulation of the plasma corticol rhythms in man. In A. Reinberg & F. Halbert (Eds) *Chronopharmacology* New York: Pergamon

Visintainer, M.A., Seligman, M.E.P., & Volpicelli, J. (1983) Helplessness, chronic stress and tumor development. *Psychosomatic Medicine*, 45, 75

Von Bertalanffy, L. (1955) An essay on the relativity of categories. *Philosophy of Science*, 22, 243-62

Von Bertalanffy, L. (1964) The mind-body problem: a new view. *Psychosomatic Medicine*, 26, 29-45

Von Bertalanffy, L. (1968) *Organismic psychology and systems theory*. Barre: Barre Publishing

Von Bonsdorff, I., et. al. (1981) Somatic diseases in mental health patients. In Achte & Pakaslahti (1981): 189-94

Waaler, H.T., & Lund, E. (1983) Association between body height and death from breast cancer. *British Journal of Cancer*, 48, 149-50

Wald, N.J., et. al. (1980) *Smoking habits among smokers of different types of cigarettes. Thorax*, 35, 925-8

Wald, N.J., et. al. (1983) Inhaling and lung cancer: an anomally explained. *British Medical Journal*, 287, 1273-5

Walter, J.B., & Israel, M.S. (1979) *General Pathology*. London: Churchill Livingstone

Wanlass, R.L., & Prinz, R.J. (1982) Methodological issues in conceptualizing and treating childhood social isolation. *Psychological Bulletin*, 92, 39-55

Weddington, W.W., Miller, N.J., & Sweet, D.L. (1984) Anticipatory nausea and vomiting associated with cancer chemotherapy. *Journal of Psychosomatic Research*, 28, 73-8

Weinberg, R.A. (1983) A molecular basis of cancer. *Scientific American*, 249, 5, 102

Weiner, H. (1982) The prospects for psychosomatic medicine. *Psychosomatic Medicine*, 44, 491-517

Weiss, S.M., et. al. (Eds) (1981) *Perspectives on Behavioural Medicine.* New York: Academic Press

Wellisch, D.K., Jamison, K.R., & Pasnau, R.O. (1978) Psychosocial aspects of mastectomy. II. The man's perspective. *American Journal of Psychiatry*, 135, 543-6

Whelan, E. (1980) *Preventing cancer.* London: Sphere

Whitehead, W.E., & Bosmajian, L. (1982) Behavioural medicine approaches to gastrointestinal disorders. *Journal of Consulting & Clinical Psychology*, 50, 972-83

Whittemore, A.S., Paffenberger, R.S., et. al. (1983) Early precursors of pancreatic cancer in college men. *Journal of Chronic Disease*, 36, 251-6

Whittemore, A.S., Paffenberger, R.S., et. al. (1984) Early precursors of urogenital cancers in former college men. *Journal of Urology*, 132, 1256-61

Wilf, R., et. al. (1983) Internal body image of the brain. *Psychotherapy & Psychosomatics*, 39, 129-35

Wilkins, J.R., Reiches, N.A., & Kruse, C.W. (1979) Organic chemical contaminants in drinking water and cancer. *American Journal of Epidemiology*, 110, 420-48

Williams, A.W., Ware, J.E., & Donald, C.A. (1981) A model of mental health, life events and social supports applicable to general populations. *Journal of Health & Social Behaviour*, 22, 324

Wilson-Barnett, J. (1984) Intervention to alleviate patient stress: a review. *Journal of Psychosomatic Research*, 28, 63-72

Wirsching, M., Druner, H.U., & Herrmann, G. (1975) Results of psychosocial adjustment to long-term colostomy. *Psychotherapy & Psychosomatics*, 26, 245-56

Wirsching, M., et. al. (1981) Breast cancer in context. In Achte (1981)

Wirsching, M., et. al. (1981) Psychological identification of breast cancer patients before biopsy. *Journal of Psychosomatic Research*, 26, 1-10

Wirsching, M., & Wirsching, B. (1980) Family dynamics and family therapy of cancer patients. *Proceedings of the 13th European Conference on Psychosomatic Research*, Istanbul

Worden, J.W., & Weisman, A.D. (1980) Do cancer patients really want counselling? *General Hospital Psychiatry*, 2, 100-3

Wortman, C.B., & Lehman, D.R. (1984) *Reactions to victims of life crises: support attempts that fail.* University of Michigan: Ann Arbor

Wynder, E.L., & Hecht, S. (Eds) (1976) *Lung cancer.* Geneva: UICC

Zimmermann, M., Drings, P., & Wagner, C. (1984) *Pain in the cancer patient.* Berlin: Springer-Verlag

Zuzunegui, M.V., et. al. (1986) Male influences on cervical cancer risk. *American Journal of Epidemiology*, 123, 302-7

Index

adolescence, 42-3, 73-4, 155-6
adult life, 43-4, 60, 74-8, 156
Africa, 103-4
alcohol, 19, 46, 60
alimentary cancers *see* digestive
    tract, cancers of
alternative medical practice, 10, 11,
    31, 39-41, 138
altruism, 109 *see also* selfishness
American Medical Association, 137
anger
    expression of, 35
    felt by cancer victims, 183-4
    suppression of, 33, 109
    see also emotions
animal studies, 31, 38-9
anti-cancer medication *see* drugs
anxiety, 27, 33, 63, 64, 84, 85, 97, 191
asbestos, 19
attitudes
    to cancer, 13-14
    to life, 38

benign growths, 15, 23, 108
bladder cancer, 18, 19, 46
body
    awareness of internal body states,
       70, 71, 127-8, 139, 140, 144-5,
       149
    coping with changes after
       surgery, 178-84

fixations, 100-1
hatred of parts of, 136
healthy functioning of, 79-80, 81
support systems, 23-7 *see also*
    central nervous system;
    endocrine or hormonal
    system; immune system
bowel cancers *see* digestive tract,
    cancers of; stoma
breast cancer
    age group at risk, 156
    case studies, 110-3, 179-81, 187
    coping with body changes after
       surgery, 178-81
    cultural factors, 21-2, 103-4
    development of breasts, 102-3
    diet, 22, 46, 105, 108, 187
    discussion of, 101-113
    function of the breasts, 103-4
    hereditary factors, 18
    hormones, 105-8
    incidence, 21, 105
    physiology of breasts, 102
    pregnancy as a protection
       against, 21-2, 105-7
    psychology, 32-3, 34, 109-113
    screening techniques, 11
    Steps 1 and 2: exposing breast to
       risk, 105-8
    Step 3: exposing breast to cancer
       growths, 108-9

surgery, 161, 162, 178-9
survivors, 34
symptoms, 105
breathing, 82, 83-4, 185-6

carcinogens
    action on cells, 23
    role in development of cancer,
        18-20, 23, 28, 29, 45, 46, 52-6,
        67-8, 83-4, 94-6, 105, 114, 129,
        130
    society's role in reducing
        exposure to, 151-2
    types of, 18-19, 46
    see also eating habits; radiation;
        sexual habits; smoking;
        sunshine, effects of
carcinomas, 16
case studies
    bowel cancer, 98-100, 182-3
    breast cancer, 110-3, 179-81, 187
    cervical cancer, 116, 117-9, 121-2
    lung cancer, 89-92
    skin cancer, 124
    smoking problem, 89-92, 141-51
    testicular cancer, 123-4
causes of cancer, 17-24 *see also* three
    steps to cancer
cells, 14, 15-16, 23
central nervous system (CNS)
    examples of working, 50, 51
    function of, 24-5
    in relation to immune system, 47,
        49, 64, 65
    role in step 2 of cancer
        development, 28, 29, 45, 46,
        47, 56-63
    mentioned, 26, 27, 44, 84, 97, 109,
        166-7
cervical cancer
    case studies, 116, 117-9, 121-2
    cultural factors, 22
    discussion of, 114-22
    drugs used in treatment, 163
    incidence of, 11, 22, 115
    Pap smear test, 22, 32, 152
    personal hygiene, 115
    psychology, 32, 120-22
    reactions to, 178
    screening techniques, 11, 22, 152
    sexual habits, 22, 46, 115, 116-7
    Step 1 risk, 114, 115-7
    Step 2 risk, 117-9
    Step 3 risk, 119-20

surgery, 178
symptoms, 114
change in status experienced by
    cancer victims, 163-4
charismatic healers, 41 *see also*
    alternative medical practice
childhood
    as vulnerable life crisis, 154-5
    cancer victims' experience in,
        31-2, 37, 42
    high risk individuals, 69-73
    immune system, 64
    normal overriding learnt, 57-8
    selfishness, 174
cholesterol levels, 36
CNS *see* central nervous system
colds, 48-50
colorectal cancer, 46, 52
connective cell tissue, 15, 16
constipation, 52, 59, 96, 98, 99, 100,
    132, 140-1
contiguous studies, 31, 33-4
cultural factors *see* social and
    cultural factors
cysts, 107-8 *see also* benign growths

danger signs
    for people at low risk, 132-3
    for people at moderate risk,
        135-6
denial of reality, 34, 168-9
diagnosis, 158, 159-60
diet *see* eating habits
digestive tract, cancers of (stomach,
    intestinal and bowel)
    age group at risk from stomach
        cancer, 156
    case studies, 98-100, 182-3
    diet, 21, 94-5
    discussion of, 92-101
    functions of digestive tract, 92-3
    incidence of stomach cancer,
        18-19, 21
    psychology, 98-101
    Step 1: exposure to carcinogens,
        94-6
    Step 2: interfering with normal
        digestive functions, 96-7
    Step 3: lowered immunity, 97-8
    surgery for bowel cancer, 162 *see
        also* stoma
    symptoms, 94
discomfort, persistent, 135-6
disorientation, 176

doctors, 13, 41, 160, 161, 163-4
dreaming, 188
drugs, 161, 162, 163, 167, 184, 186

East Anglia, 18
eating habits
    bowel cancer in relation to, 95
    breast cancer in relation to, 22,
      46, 105, 108
    colorectal cancer in relation to,
      46, 52
    food and drug scrutinizing
      agencies, 151
    modifying, 137, 186-7
    psychological aspects, 54, 55-6,
      59, 95, 96, 108
    stomach cancer in relation to, 21,
      94-5
Egypt, 18, 19
emotions
    attitudes learnt in childhood, 42,
      70-1, 174
    inability to express, 32, 35, 36, 44,
      62, 70-1, 87, 109, 133, 140, 170
    learning to express, 148-50, 193
    rest-activity cycles, 60-1
    see also anger; repressive
      personalities
endocrine or hormonal system
    examples of working, 50, 51
    functions, 25-6
    in relation to immune system, 47,
      49
    role in Step 2 of cancer
      development, 28, 29, 45, 56-63
    mentioned, 27, 44, 97
epithelium cell tissue, 15, 16
evacuation of waste, 187-8 *see also*
    constipation
exercise, 188

faith, 172
family, friends and relatives, coping
    with, 173-5
Far East, 21, 105
fatigue, 38, 44, 74, 131, 133, 136
fatty foods, 22, 95
fibre, 95
fighting cancer, 34, 168, 169, 189
follow-up medical action, 161-3
foodstuffs *see* eating habits
freezing of emotional reactions (in
    shock), 176
Freudian theories, 10, 30

geographical factors, 18-19
green vegetables, 95
growths, 14-17

habits, bad
    in high-risk individuals, 139, 140,
      142-4
    in low-risk individuals, 131, 132,
      133, 135
    in moderate-risk individuals,
      135, 137
    making people aware of, 152-3
    need for cancer victims to
      change, 163, 169, 185-8
Harvard-Pennsylvania study, 35, 36
healthy body function, 79-80, 81
helplessness, feelings of, 33, 34, 43,
    44, 66, 74, 88
heredity, 17-18
high-risk individuals
    preventive strategy for, 139-51
    psychology, 68-78, 130, 152
Hodgkins' Disease, 36, 42
hope, psychology of, 190-1
hopelessness, feelings of, 32, 33, 34,
    35
hormonal system *see* endocrine or
    hormonal system
hormones and the breast, 105-8
hostility, feelings of, 183-4
hypnotism, 41

images, use of, 190-1
immune system
    cancer patients, 185, 186
    function, 24, 26
    role in Step 3 of cancer
      development, 28-9, 45, 47,
      48-50, 63-6, 67, 87-9, 97-8,
      109, 119, 167
    vulnerability, 27
    mentioned, 36, 44, 129, 152
industrialization, 19, 20
intermediate growths, 15
internal body states, awareness of,
    70, 71, 127-8, 139, 140, 144-5, 149
interpersonal sensitivity, 63-4
intestinal cancer *see* digestive tract,
    cancers of

Japan, 21, 97, 103
Johns Hopkins University study, 36-8

Kansas study, 35, 36

King's College Hospital, London, 34
Kissen, D.M., 31-2

Le Shan, L., 32, 38
leukaemias, 16, 42, 156, 162, 163
life crises, 154-7
lip cancers, 18, 124 *see also* skin
  cancer
liver cancer, 46
loneliness, 64, 120
low-risk individuals, 130-5
lung cancer
  age group at risk, 156
  breathing patterns, 82, 83-4
  case studies, 87-8, 89-92
  discussion of, 81-92
  incidence, 11, 20, 21
  psychology, 31-2, 89-92
  smoking, 18, 20-1, 36, 46, 52, 82,
    83, 84, 85, 86, 88, 89, 90, 91,
    92, 185
  Step 1: exposure to carcinogens,
    83-4
  Step 2: overriding the body's
    normal response, 84-7
  Step 3: lowered immunity, 87-9
  symptoms, 81
lymph cells, 15, 16
lymphomas, 16, 42, 156

Magarey, Christopher, 40-1
male reproductive organs *see*
    testicles, cancer of
Manchester University study, 108
mastectomy, 34 *see also* breast
    cancer
masturbation, 123
medical action, 160-1 *see also* drugs;
    follow-up medical action;
    radiation treatment; surgery
moderate-risk individuals, 135-8

natural killer cell activity (NKCA),
    63, 64, 65, 67
nervous tension, 37-8, 97, 136
nicotine *see* smoking
NKCA *see* natural killer cell activity
nursing staff, 13, 163-4

obsessional behaviour, 37, 44, 64
occupational risks, 19
old age, 156
overriding
  cancer in relation to, 60-3, 66, 67,

    84-7, 97, 107, 108, 131, 152,
    166-7
  discussion of, 56-63
  faulty, 58-60, 61-3
  normal, 57-8
  types of, 56-7
overweight, 27

pain, 17
pancreatic cancer, 125
Pap smear test, 22, 32, 152
parent-child relationships, 37, 42,
    43, 64, 70-1, 72, 73-4, 156
penis, cancer of *see* testicles, cancer
    of
personal hygiene, 115-6, 123
personality and cancer, 30-44
  animal studies, 31, 38-9
  contiguous studies, 31, 33-4
  prospective studies, 31, 34-8
  retrospective studies, 31-3
  summary of characteristics
    predisposing individuals to
    cancer, 42-4
  unorthodox medical
    practitioners, 31, 39-41
pollution, 151
polyposis coli, 17-18
pregnancy, 21-2, 102-3, 104, 105-7
prevention of cancer, 126-57
  high-risk individuals, 139-51
  low-risk individuals, 130-5
  moderate-risk individuals, 135-8
  recognizing interplay between
    mind and body, 126-8
  society's role in, 151-4
  vulnerable life crises, 154-7
preventive strategy for high-risk
    individuals, 139-51
  Step 1: modifying habits, 139,
    140, 142-4
  Step 2: attending to body sounds,
    139, 140, 144-5
  Step 3: giving yourself time, 139,
    140, 141, 145-6
  Step 4: improving target organ's
    functioning, 139, 141, 146-7
  Step 5: improving relationships,
    139, 141, 147-50
  Step 6: coping with stress, 139,
    150-1
prospective studies, 31, 34-8
psychological coping patterns,
    changing, 188-92

psychological help, 78, 153, 192, 195
psychology of cancer
  common cancers, 79-125
  developing a new psychology,
    45-78
  historical review, 9-11, 30-1
  personality and cancer, 30-44
  preventing cancer, 126-57
  surviving cancer, 158-93
  understanding cancer, 13-29

radiation, 19, 46, 151 *see also*
  sunshine, effects of
radiation treatment, 162, 167
recovery from shock, 177
regression, 176-7
Reich, Wilhelm, 10
relationships
  cancer prevention and, 139,
    147-50
  dependence on, 133-4
  high-risk individuals and, 75-8,
    139, 141, 147-50
  importance in survival from
    cancer, 170-3, 192
  parent-child, 37, 42, 43, 64, 70-1,
    72, 73-4, 156
  radical, 77-8
  research work, 32, 33, 38, 42, 43,
    109
  status-quo maintaining, 75-6
  supportive, 76-7
religious belief, 172
repressive personalities, 30, 31, 36,
  52 *see also* emotions
reproductive system, cancers of,
  114-24 *see also* cervical cancer;
  testicles, cancer of
research findings on psychology of
  cancer, 10, 30-44
rest-activity cycles, 60-1
retinoblastoma, 18, 125
retirement, 156
retrospective studies, 31-3
revulsion, feelings of, 178, 179, 180

sarcomas, 16
scars, 178, 179, 180, 181
screening techniques, 11, 22, 152
selfishness, 172-3, 173-5, 186
sexual habits, 22, 46, 55, 114, 115,
  116, 123, 137 *see also* sexual
    intercourse
sexual intercourse

attitudes to, 117, 120, 122
cancer victims and, 179-81,
  182-3, 188
see also sexual habits
shock, coping with, 175-7
side effects of treatment, 162-3, 165,
  166, 184
Simonton clinic, 40, 190-1
skin cancers, 16, 18, 46, 52, 124-5
sleep, 27, 188
smoking
  campaign against, 151, 152
  case studies, 89-92, 141-51
  changing habits, 137, 152, 185,
    186
  cultural approval of, 20-1, 53, 55,
    85
  in relation to lung cancer, 18,
    20-1, 36, 46, 52, 82, 83, 84, 85,
    86, 88, 89, 90, 91, 92, 185
  patterns of, 53, 85-6
  psychological aspects, 53-4, 60,
    85, 86, 89, 90, 91, 100, 132
  three steps to cancer model
    illustrated in relation to, 46-7
social and cultural factors, 20-2,
  53-5, 103-4
society's role in cancer prevention,
  151-4
soil conditions, 18-19
South America, 95, 105
spontaneous remission of cancer, 39
stamina, lack of *see* fatigue
stoma, 162, 181-3
stomach cancer *see* digestive tract,
  cancers of
stress
  animal studies, 39
  cholesterol levels, 35-6
  coping with, 101, 139, 150-1, 154,
    175
  high-risk individuals, 43, 73, 74,
    139, 150-1
  immune system affected by, 27,
    63, 64, 66
sugar, 22, 46, 108
sunshine, effects of, 16, 17, 18, 19,
  46, 52, 53, 124
surgery, 9, 161, 162, 170-1
  coping with body changes after,
    178-84
survival, psychology of, 169-93
  task 1: building supporting
    relationships, 170-3

task 2: coping with family, friends and relatives, 173-5
task 3: coping with shock, 175-7
task 4: coping with body changes, 178-84
task 5: changing bad habits, 185-8
task 6: changing psychological coping patterns, 188-92
task 7: directing your own survival, 192-3
surviving cancer, 10, 33-4, 158-93
how to think about having cancer, 165-9
psychology of survival, 169-93
research, 10, 33-4, 168-9
response to diagnosis, 158, 159
what having cancer means, 159-64
survivors, cancer, 10, 33-4, 168-9
Switzerland, 18

tension, 37-8, 97, 136
testicles, cancer of, 22, 46, 122-4
Thames water, 20
thinking positively about cancer, 165-9
finding time, 166
reactions to disease, 165-6
thinking about what can be done, 166-8
who survives cancer, 168-9
Thomas, Dr. C.B., study by, 36-8
three steps to cancer, 28-9, 45-68, 129
as shown in particular types of cancer *see* type of cancer
how to think about, 48-52
Step 1: presence of carcinogens, 28, 29, 45, 46, 52-6, 67, 68, 129
Step 2: central nervous and endocrine factors, 28, 29, 45, 46-7, 50-1, 56-63, 67, 68, 129
Step 3: failure of immune system, 28-9, 45, 47, 48-50, 63-6, 67, 68
see also causes of cancer
throat cancer, 46
thyroid cancers, 18
time, importance of
for cancer victims, 166
for high-risk individuals, 71-2, 139, 145-6
tumours *see* growths

ulcerative colitis, 100-1
understanding cancer, 13-29
attitudes, 13-14
body's support systems, 24-7
causes, 17-24
growths, 14-17
see also three steps to cancer
unorthodox or alternative medical practitioners, 10, 11, 31, 39-41, 138
United States, 105

viral infection in relation to cervical cancer, 114, 115
vulnerable life crises, 154-7

Wales, North, 18
warning signs, 137
water, drinking, 19-20

xeroderma pigmentosum, 17

Yugoslav study, 35-6